Special Care Programs for People with Dementia

Special Care Programs for People with Dementia

Edited by
Stephanie B. Hoffman, Ph.D.
Mary Kaplan, M.S.W.

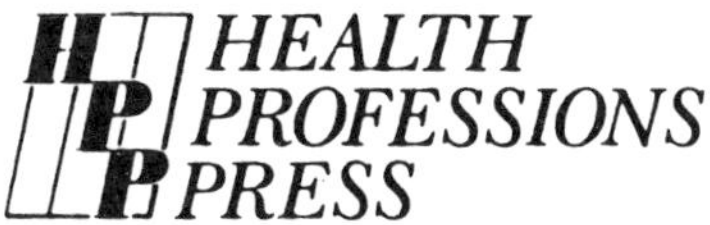

Baltimore • London • Toronto • Sydney

Health Professions Press, Inc.
Post Office Box 10624
Baltimore, Maryland 21285-0624

Typeset by PRO-IMAGE Corporation, York, Pennsylvania.
Manufactured in the United States of America by
The Maple Press Company, York, Pennsylvania.

Library of Congress Cataloging-in-Publication Data

Special care programs for people with dementia / edited by Stephanie B. Hoffman, Mary Kaplan.
p. cm.
Includes bibliograpical references and index.
ISBN 1-878812-33-5
1. Dementia—Patients—Nursing home care—United States.
I. Hoffman, Stephanie B. II. Kaplan, Mary.
[DNLM: 1. Dementia. Senile—therapy. 2. Long-Term Care.
3. Skilled Nursing Facilities. WT 155 S741 1996]
RC521.S647 1996
362.1'9683–dc20
DNLM/DLC
for Library of Congress 96-14721
CIP

British Library Cataloguing in Publication Data are available from the British Library.

Contents

About the Editors

Stephanie B. Hoffman is the director of Interdisciplinary Team Training and Primary Care Education at the James A. Haley Veterans Hospital in Tampa, Florida. She serves on the Faculty Advisory Council of the University of South Florida Institute on Aging, and as a coordinator for regional and national conferences on dementia. She received a master's degree in Clinical Gerontology and a doctorate in Human Development and Family Studies from Pennsylvania State University.

A life span developmental psychologist, Dr. Hoffman has worked in the field of geriatrics/gerontology for over 15 years. She has received funded grants to study the communication and management aspects of dementia. At the James A. Haley Veterans Hospital she has trained students and staff in the following disciplines: nursing, medicine, psychiatry, psychology, pharmacy, podiatry, social work, speech-language pathology, audiology, occupational therapy, dietetics, physical therapy, and chaplain services.

Dr. Hoffman has conducted workshops on dementia management and team training throughout the United States for continuing education programs and long-term care and other settings. She has published in the areas of geropsychology, dementia, team building, and nonverbal communication, and coauthored (with C.A. Platt) the book *Comforting the Confused: Strategies for Managing Dementia*, published by Springer Publishing in 1991.

Mary Kaplan is a consultant on aging programs, dementia care, and case management services for health care organizations. She teaches in the Department of Gerontology at the University of South Florida. Ms. Kaplan received her master's degree in social work from Catholic University, and is a Florida state licensed clinical social worker and a member of the Academy of Certified Social Workers, National Association of Social Workers.

Ms. Kaplan has over 20 years of experience in the aging and health care fields as a direct care service provider, administrator, and educator. As past Education Coordinator for the Tampa Bay, Florida Chapter of the Alzheimer's Association, Ms. Kaplan provided training in dementia care for aging program staff in a three-county area.

She has written numerous articles for professional journals and book chapters on aging issues, and is the author of *Clinical Practice with Families of Dementia Patients*, published by Taylor & Francis in 1996.

Contributors

Mary Guerriero Austrom, Ph.D.
Department of Psychiatry and the Indiana Alzheimer's Disease Center
Indiana University School of Medicine
Clinical Building 279
541 Clinical Drive
Indianapolis, IN 46202-5111

Edna L. Ballard, A.C.S.W., C.M.S.W.
Duke University Medical Center
Box 3600
Busse Building, Room 3510
Durham, NC 27710

Kathleen C. Buckwalter, Ph.D., R.N., F.A.A.N.
College of Nursing, 444 NB
University of Iowa
Iowa City, IA 52242

Susan G. Cooley, Ph.D.
U.S. Department of Veterans Affairs
Office of Geriatrics and Extended Care
810 Vermont Avenue, NW
Washington, DC 20420

Lucia K. DeBauge, M.Arch., Ph.D.
Senior Design of Texas
1224 Cliffview Drive
Waco, TX 76710-4290
Baylor University
Waco, TX 76798

Dani Fallin, B.S.
Roskamp Laboratories
Psychiatry & Behavior Medicine
TGH Psychiatry Center, MDC-14
3515 East Fletcher Avenue
Tampa, FL 33613

Linda A. Gerdner, M.A., R.N.
College of Nursing
University of Iowa
Iowa City, IA 52242

Jerry Gilmer, Ph.D.
College of Nursing
University of Iowa
Iowa City, IA 52242

Marsha E. Goodwin-Beck, R.N.-C., M.A., M.S.N.
U.S. Department of Veterans Affairs
Office of Geriatrics and Extended Care
810 Vermont Avenue, NW
Washington, DC 20420

Geri R. Hall, M.A., R.N.
College of Nursing
University of Iowa
Iowa City, IA 52242

Gail Harbour, R.N.
230 Grandview Street
Bennington, VT 05201

Jonathan B. Hoyne, B.A.
Roskamp Laboratories
Psychiatry & Behavior Medicine
TGH Psychiatry Center, MDC-14
3515 East Fletcher Avenue
Tampa, FL 33613

David A. Lindeman, Ph.D.
Rush-Presbyterian-St. Luke's Medical Center
Departments of Neurological Sciences and Internal Medicine
1645 West Jackson Boulevard, Suite 675
Chicago, IL 60612

Michael J. Mullan, M.D., Ph.D., M.R.C.Psych.
Roskamp Laboratories
Psychiatry & Behavior Medicine
TGH Psychiatry Center, MDC-14
3515 East Fletcher Avenue
Tampa, FL 33613

Sylvia Nissenboim, A.C.S.W.
Geri-Active Consultants
9518 Engel Lane
St. Louis, MO 63132

Philip D. Sloane, M.D., M.P.H.
Department of Family Medicine
University of North Carolina at Chapel Hill
Manning Drive, Campus Box 7595
Chapel Hill, NC 27599-7595

Toni Tripp-Reimer, Ph.D., F.A.A.N.
College of Nursing
University of Iowa
Iowa City, IA 52242

Ladislav Volicer, M.D., Ph.D.
Edith Nourse Rogers Memorial Veterans Hospital
200 Springs Road
Bedford, MA 01750
Boston University School of Medicine
Boston, MA 02118

Bonnie Wakefield, M.A., R.N.
College of Nursing
University of Iowa
Iowa City, IA 52242

James A. Waterman, M.S.N., R.N.
College of Nursing
University of Iowa
Iowa City, IA 52242

Foreword

With the aging of the American population, the numbers of older people with dementia are increasing. Although most people with dementia are cared for in the home or within the community, when their needs become overwhelming or family assistance is no longer available, nursing facilities become the settings in which many of these older people live their final days. In the early 1990s policy makers, health care administrators, and researchers began asking questions such as the following about the quality of care for people with dementia in nursing facilities: Are the existing care policies and programs designed to meet the needs of physically frail older adults? Do they adequately ensure institutionally based programs that provide high-quality care for people with dementia? Are they simply a marketing tool to enhance the revenue of nursing facilities? Concern about the quality of care for residents with dementia has spawned the special care unit movement, and subsequently, evaluation of unit effectiveness.

The answers to these care questions are only beginning to emerge. Although definitive answers are not expected until the end of the 1990s, the literature, which summarizes the state of knowledge and identifies major research directions related to special care programs, is expanding rapidly. In particular, three synthesizing activities that have provided impetus to the field are worth highlighting: 1) the 1990 conference, "Special Care Units for Alzheimer's Disease: Innovations in Long-Term Care," which was reported on by Berg, Buckwalter, and Chafetz in their article "Special Care Units for Persons with Dementia," published in 1991 in the *Journal of the American Geriatrics Society*; 2) the 1992 Office of Technology Assessment report, *Special Care for People with Alzheimer's and Reimbursement Issues*; and 3) the 1994 *Alzheimer's Disease and Associated Disorders* supplemental volume, *Special Dementia Care: Research, Policy, and Practice Issues.*

Special care programs for people with dementia are rapidly proliferating in the United States. Over 1,500 units have been established in nursing facilities and many others are in the planning stages. With this rate of growth and with the passing of the first half of the 1990s, it is wise to revisit the clinical, research, and policy issues involved in developing and evaluating special care programs. The 1995 conference, "Dementia Specific Care Units: Winning Strategies for Success," from which this volume is derived, provided an excellent mid-decade forum for reviewing current issues and stressed practical solutions for improving care of people with Alzheimer's disease.

What can we expect by the end of the 1990s? Will there be a greater proliferation of special care programs in nursing facilities? What will the programs look like? A mid-decade census of specialty nursing facility care is now underway, which will provide an update from the 1990–1991 national profile. It is likely that diversity in and evolution of special care will continue, with differentiation of special care programs according to disease progression. Special care for people with dementia is also moving out of the nursing facility and into other care settings, such as assisted living facilities.

By the year 2000, definitive findings from the National Institute on Aging's (NIA) Collaborative Studies of Special Care Units for Alzheimer's Disease[1] will become available from the 10 individual research sites involved as well as from cross-site analyses. These studies are examining the critical questions posed by family members, health care administrators, and policy makers, such as the following:

- How does care provided in special care units differ from that provided in regular units in nursing facilities? Can differences be noted in residents' physical conditions, psychological conditions, or social behaviors?
- Does family involvement increase when relatives with dementia are placed in special care programs rather than in regular care?
- How do special care programs influence the abilities of administrators to track and monitor the quality of nursing care in light of new federal guidelines (e.g., Omnibus Budget Reconciliation Act of 1987 and 1990) concerning nursing facilities?
- In what ways do special care programs benefit residents without dementia?
- What is the cost–benefit ratio?

Although each of the 10 NIA studies has unique features, investigators from each study collaborate on issues such as defining what constitutes a special care program, determining how residents with and without de-

[1]For further information on the NIA's special care program initiative, contact Marcia Ory, BSR/NIA/NIH, Gateway Building, Suite 533, Bethesda, Maryland 20892.

mentia will be identified, and evaluating how care in special care programs affects the residents, staff, and family caregivers. The NIA special care program initiative has two goals: 1) to determine whether and how special care programs improve the quality of care provided to residents with dementia and their families and 2) to provide public policy makers with the necessary information to facilitate the decision-making process, particularly with regard to regulatory and reimbursement issues.

Contrary to the simplistic notions of the past, special care programs are neither monolithic entities nor are they static. To avoid simple, perhaps flawed, notions about the merits of special care programs, it is necessary to identify and evaluate different components of care (e.g., special programming, staffing, environmental modifications). One anticipated benefit from the NIA initiative is advances in state-of-the-art measurement and research designs for studying people with cognitive impairment in nursing facilities. These advances may involve, for example, a merging of research on dementia and nursing facility studies with research from mainstream disciplines in order to develop new measures and longitudinal analyses for assessing changes in dementia-related behaviors over time.

Progress in research will also come with greater attention paid to the importance of subgroup analyses and targeting approaches. Although special care programs will be evaluated initially for the general impact they have on systems and people, it is much more likely that specific aspects of special care will have particular benefits for individuals with specific behavioral or functional problems. For example, is a special care program required to offer all recommended parameters of care in order to achieve benefits, or might attention focused on staff training issues produce benefits for residents with early-stage dementia and their caregivers? Similarly, as the United States becomes increasingly culturally diverse, there will need to be a greater recognition of the impact of different ethnic groups on resident experiences, resident care preferences, and administrative–staff–resident interactions in special care versus traditional care.

Some people have called for greater regulation of special care programs to ensure that consumers actually receive "specialized" care. However, a review of the research (although disclosing much diversity in what is labeled "special care") suggests that widespread adoption of a strict regulatory approach would be premature and may actually stifle the development of care-enhancing innovations. To this end, researchers have been more supportive of a program disclosure or guideline approach.

What will the future bring? Beds in special care units account for approximately 10% of the available beds in certified nursing facilities. If these programs are found to be beneficial, will proliferation accelerate? What is the true meaning of "specialized care" when approximately 70% of nursing home residents are estimated to have some level of cognitive impairment? One of the most positive legacies of the special care movement may be the provision of insight into how care can be enhanced for all residents of nursing facilities. In this scenario, "specialized care" will be synonymous with "high-quality care," which is the goal of the initial inquiries into the development and effectiveness of special care for people with dementia. Concern about the care provided in nursing facilities will continue to be addressed by the Workgroup on Research and Evaluation in Special Care Units (WRESCU),[2] a national workgroup of more than 100 people interested in special care programs for people with dementia in both institutional and residential settings.

It is difficult to predict the future other than in very broad brushstrokes. The James A. Haley Veterans' Hospital, Menorah Manor, and the Tampa-St. Petersburg Alzheimer's Association chapter are to be commended for organizing the stimulating and provocative conference from which this volume is derived. *Special Care Programs for People with Dementia* provides concrete examples of special care programs and suggests how practitioners and administrators can design care settings to achieve goals for high-quality care for residents with dementia and their caregivers. The volume is especially valuable for translating emergent research findings into everyday care strategies that can make an immediate difference in the lives of individuals with dementia and their caregivers. Researchers continue to debate the precise definition of special care programs, the consequences of different parameters of care, and the effects of that care on different types of residents and caregivers. This volume helps define the major care issues and provides practical strategies for practitioners and administrators who are responsible for the care of people with dementia.

Marcia G. Ory, Ph.D., M.P.H.
National Institute on Aging

REFERENCES

Berg, L., Buckwalter, K.C., & Chafetz, P.K. (1991). Special care units for persons with dementia. *Journal of the American Geriatric Society, 39*, 1229–1236.

Holmes, D., Ory, M., & Teresi, J. (1994). Special care units: An overview of research, program and policy perspectives. *Alzheimer's Disease and Associated Disorders: An International Journal, 8*(Suppl. 1), S5–S13.

Office of Technology Assessment. (1992). *Special care for people with Alzheimer's and other dementias: Consumer education, research, regulatory, and reimbursement issues*. Washington, DC: U.S. Government Printing Office.

[2]For further information on WRESCU, contact D. Holmes, Hebrew Home for the Aged at Riverdale, 5901 Palisade Avenue, Riverdale, New York 10471.

Preface

This book was a labor of commitment and respect—respect for the knowledge, creativity, and professionalism of our contributors, and beyond that, respect for the struggles and challenges of people with dementia.

A resident in a good special care unit wrote the following note to his wife on the week he was admitted to the unit:

Dear Esther,

Just to let you know that I am in trouble + I have been robbed. I don't have 1¢ in my pockets. I doubt that I will be able to get this letter out. It is impossible for me to get out. This is prisson (sic) make no misstake (sic).

Please try to help me!!

Stan

This resident makes a telling statement. Special care units can feel like prison. Residents often feel robbed of their familiar environments, their possessions and money, and their freedom. As a result, we have a special responsibility to develop programs and environments that nurture rather than restrict.

We know that the profit motive often drives the development of innovations in any field. However, it seems to us that in this caregiving field innovations are also derived from the desire to help. In the development of this book, we were motivated to help improve the quality of life for people with dementia and the people striving to take care of them.

The environments we create can cause increased despair for people with cognitive losses or they can buffer those losses and shore up waning dignity. This book is a guide for improving the quality of unit design and care strategies. The book contains the best ideas of caring professionals for very special programs, designs, and solutions that will enhance our clients' lives. Many of these ideas and suggestions have been and continue to be carefully researched. They are guidelines for success in your efforts to develop special care programs for people with dementia.

Special Care Programs for People with Dementia

1

Special Care Programs
Challenges to Success

Mary Kaplan, M.S.W.

Although there has been tremendous growth in the number of special care programs in recent years, there is a scarcity of information about the problems encountered by administrators, program directors, and other professionals in the operation of these programs and the provision of services to people with dementia. Much of the current research on dementia-specific care has focused on the effects, most often positive, of special care programs on participants, residents, and caregivers. Although this is certainly an important area for research, there is also a need for systematic information to be furnished to dementia care providers who are faced with a confusing array of policy and procedural issues.

In 1995 a survey conducted at a conference, *Dementia Specific Care Units: Winning Strategies for Success*, attempted to identify the challenges involved in the implementation of special care programs, as well as some of the innovations that had proved successful for individual facilities. A total of 58 conference participants who were involved in the operation or coordination of special care programs in the United States and Canada responded to the survey. Although this survey sample does not claim to be representative of all providers of dementia care, it does provide some insight into the problems they are facing.

Table 1.1 lists the ten most frequently reported problems identified by survey respondents. This chapter addresses these problems and examines additional issues of concern in the provision of care to people with dementia.

PHYSICAL ENVIRONMENT

The greatest challenge in the provision of dementia care expressed by survey respondents (64%) was the physical environment. Complaints most frequently cited were institutional settings, lack of secured outside areas, and units that were too small to allow for resident traffic and special programs. Dementia-specific care facilities are often limited by state and fire regulations in their attempts to modify the existing environment to meet the needs of the person with dementia. This was particularly true for skilled nursing facilities that are regulated in accordance with a medical model.

More Homelike Setting

A common complaint is that the physical environment of many special care programs is too institutional and does not provide a homelike atmosphere. Many health care facilities use existing space to house dementia programs. Although these environments tend to be sterile and uninviting, touches can be added to create a homelike atmosphere without great expense.

The following suggestions can be helpful:

1. Replace hard, shiny tile or linoleum with cushioned vinyl or carpeting that is specially designed for use in health care facilities.
2. Use texture in upholstery, drapes, and wall hangings.
3. Select a color scheme and furniture that contribute to a traditional decor, like that found in residents' homes.
4. Replace institutional fluorescent lighting with traditional home lighting, including suspended fixtures and decorative wall sconces.
5. Add nontoxic plants, fish tanks, and birdcages that are out of residents' reach and can be easily viewed by nonambulatory as well as ambulatory residents.
6. Encourage residents' use of personal items, such as furniture, pictures, quilts, and knickknacks.
7. Use music and smells (e.g., baking, cooking) to promote feelings and memories associated with home.

Secured Outdoor Area

For many providers of dementia care, the lack of a secured outdoor area limits the opportunity for residents to wander safely and enjoy the benefits

Table 1.1. Problems identified in the operation of special care programs ($N = 58$)

Problem	Occurrence (%)
Physical environment/design	64
Inadequate programming for residents	62
Inadequate certified nursing assistant staffing	52
Lack of training for staff	43
Inadequate staffing by other types of staff	36
Inadequate funding for dementia program	33
Lack of support from facility administration	28
High staff turnover	24
Lack of opportunity for staff to attend training programs	21
Inadequate admission criteria	19

of freedom, exercise, and fresh air. If possible all special care programs should incorporate secured outdoor areas in their building plans. In addition to providing opportunities for stimulation, socializing, and activities such as gardening and outdoor sports, these areas can be used effectively for residents who pace and wander.

Ideas such as the following can be incorporated in the building plan:

1. Enclose a courtyard and allow easy access for residents to wander freely and safely. Create a wandering path with nontoxic gardens and shaded seating areas.
2. Create indoor gardens if it is not possible to plan a secured outdoor area. Play tapes of outdoor sounds, such as birds singing and water flowing.
3. Design hallways as wandering paths, with activity alcoves, plants, and rest areas.

Layout that Maximizes Privacy and Orientation

People with dementia are confused and often overwhelmed by immense space and unmanageable settings. The layouts of many traditional health care facilities feature large multipurpose rooms and dead end hallways, which can add to residents' confusion.

The following suggestions can help maximize residents' comfort:

1. Provide space in the environment that facilitates socialization (Kenshalo, 1977). The creation of small activity and seating areas helps to break up large spaces and invites the opportunity for friendship and privacy.
2. Use partitions or folding walls as barriers to divide a large area into several self-contained activity or dining areas.

3. Use paint, signs, and decorations to disguise exit doors that are off-limits to residents and to provide direction to help residents to return to a central area.
4. Use landmarks (e.g., plant, picture, personal objects) to identify residents' rooms. Color codes and signs can be used to assist residents in locating key areas.

Space for Special Programs or Activities

Special care programs should provide a sense of community to residents, enabling them to maintain daily routines and interests and encouraging them to interact with others in meaningful activities. Often, program administrators are concerned about utilizing space for as many beds as possible for maximum reimbursement and may be reluctant to allocate extra space for activities and socialization. This approach can result in increased resident problem behaviors as a result of congested central areas, high noise levels, a lack of a quiet area for agitated residents, and residents' inability to direct their energy toward meaningful activities. Environmental designs that require residents to leave the living area or to travel long distances for meals and activities should be avoided because they may increase confusion and agitation in some residents.

The following steps can be considered:

1. Reduce the number of residents in the program to create more traffic space and less congestion.
2. Convert one or two large resident rooms into an activity room or a quiet room.
3. Reduce the noise level by eliminating the public address system and limiting visitor traffic.
4. Arrange to take small groups of higher-functioning residents out of the living area for exercise and activities.

Additional information on environmental/interior design issues can be found in Chapter 8.

PROGRAMMING

Programming was found to be a major challenge to dementia care professionals, according to survey respondents. Inadequate programming for residents was the second most common problem reported (62%), and inadequate funding for programming was rated sixth (33%).

The "bricks and mortar" (construction costs involved in the building or renovation of special care programs represent a major portion of the program budget and are often referred to as the "bricks and mortar" of the program) argument has often been used to explain why the expense of building a facility prohibits expenditures for additional staff and special programming. These "extras" are not considered reimbursable through government or private insurance, and their importance is often overlooked in the development of special care programs.

Planning activities that meet the needs of residents who are in different stages of dementing illnesses can be difficult. Problem behaviors and differences in cognitive and physical functioning make it necessary to plan and conduct several types of activities.

The difference between a special care unit and a special care program is the word *program.* A facility can make modifications in an existing environment or construct a new wing or building and call it a special care unit. However, creating a special care program involves much more than designing a physical environment for people with dementia. The therapeutic program must also meet the needs of the residents, and a trained staff is required to implement the program.

Programming suggestions include the following:

1. Activity therapy for a special care program can be improved by hiring staff who are trained to work with people who have memory loss and cognitive impairment. It is important to hire an activity therapist specifically dedicated to a special care program. In nursing facilities, activities must be provided 7 days per week; an additional person who is also trained to work in the special care program must be assigned to cover early evenings, weekends, and other times when the full-time activity therapist is off.
2. By using the social instead of the medical model of care, the traditional lines of responsibility and territory of staff can be blurred to meet both the psychosocial needs and the medical needs of residents. When additional program funding is limited, nursing assistants can be trained to facilitate resident activities and to incorporate activities into resident care routines. It is important to note that this approach is recommended only in situations in which there is adequate certified nursing assistant staff (a ratio of 1:6, one staff person responsible for the care of no more than six residents [Office of Technology Assessment, 1987]).
3. The cognitive and physical functional levels of residents with dementia can be identified by using reliable measures of assessment, such as the Clinical Dementia Rating (Berg, 1984, 1988; Hughes, Berg, Danziger, Cohen, & Martin, 1982) and the Global Deterioration Scale (Reisberg, Ferris, deLeon, & Crook, 1982). Programs that provide activities and services that correspond to the levels of program participants can then be developed.
4. Specially selected music and videotapes can be used for quiet times during the day and in the evening for residents who have irregular sleep patterns. Used in combination with other activities, music and videotapes can be set up by any member of the staff or by a volunteer.
5. Volunteers can be used effectively to supplement, but not substitute for, program staff. Assisting with activities, providing an opportunity for socialization for residents, and helping staff with clerical tasks are examples of ways in which volunteers can be of service in a special

care program. Volunteers can be recruited from families, the community, religious groups, and students. It is important that all volunteers who interact with residents in a special care program be carefully screened and be required to complete dementia care training. This training should be geared toward laypersons and should include basic information on dementia and on communication techniques and approaches to managing the challenging behaviors that are common in people with dementia (The Brookdale Foundation, 1991; Kaplan & Parr, 1995).

STAFF ISSUES

Staff are an essential component of special care programs. Adequate staffing contributes to the morale and longevity of the dementia care team. Selecting a good staff and training them in the care of residents with dementia is an important first step in building a special care program. Also crucial to the success of a program is providing the support needed to help the staff continually respond to the demands of caring for residents with dementia (Kaplan, 1996; Smith, 1995).

It is not surprising that staff issues were cited several times as a problem area by survey respondents: inadequate certified nursing assistant staffing (ranked 3rd; 52%); lack of training for staff (ranked 4th; 43%); inadequate staffing by other types of staff (ranked 5th; 36%); high staff turnover (ranked 8th; 24%); and lack of opportunity for staff to attend training programs (ranked 9th; 19%). For examination purposes, staff issues are divided here into two areas of concern: adequate staff and adequate staff training.

Adequate Staff

Many facilities have not increased staff in response to the heavy care demands of residents with dementia. Individualized care provided by a consistent team of trained staff is the key to a successful special care program. Although an exact staffing pattern for specialized dementia care has not been established, the ratio of staff to residents in selected model programs is no more than 1:6 (Office of Technology Assessment, 1987). Staffing patterns should take into account the severity of dementia, physical disabilities, behavior problems, and medical problems of the residents, in addition to the environment/design of the living area. An increase in the level of staff should be considered in establishing a special care program.

Consistency of staff in a special care program helps to provide an atmosphere in which trust can be built and resident fears are diminished. Staff who are familiar with the program's philosophy and approach to care and who know the residents are able to provide a consistent daily routine; to identify changes in a resident's condition; and to create close relationships with residents, other team members, and family members.

Often, staff are "floated" to the special care program from other parts of the facility or are brought in from outside agencies. In most cases these staff are not familiar with the residents and have not been trained in dementia care.

High staff turnover and lack of staff consistency can lead to team disorganization and can produce problem behavior patterns in staff, such as manipulating or mistreating other team members, refusing to use special approaches in providing care to residents, not carrying out job responsibilities, and abusing or neglecting residents.

The following suggestions should be considered:

1. Staff should be recruited specifically for the special care program and should be selected for their experience with and commitment to the unique demands of caring for people with dementia.
2. The use of staff from other areas of the facility ("floaters") and from outside agencies should be discouraged. A dementia float pool is one solution to the common problem of maintaining a consistent, trained staff, despite periods of low staffing as a result of turnover and vacation and sick time. The pool should include both in-house staff and nurses in the community who have been trained in the care of people with dementia, are familiar with the program's residents and philosophy, and are available on an as-needed basis.
3. Staff care responsibilities should be evaluated by conducting time studies, looking at acuity levels and behaviors of residents and staff: resident ratios. The amount of time required by staff to supervise and direct residents with dementia should be considered, as well as the time spent in providing direct care. Negotiation among staff on different shifts should be encouraged to help determine ways to distribute resident care responsibilities equally by rescheduling resident care activities (e.g., if the day shift has a large number of residents that require feeding assistance, some residents' bathing might be rescheduled from morning to evening).
4. Program leadership must be clearly defined and empowered to make decisions regarding staff and program issues. The program director must have good interpersonal skills, as well as knowledge of the care of people with dementia.
5. Problem staff behavior can be averted through intense orientation efforts that provide a clear understanding of the program's goals and team roles.
6. Regularly scheduled group meetings can provide a forum for staff problem identification and resolution. The selection by team members of one or more process analyzers may be helpful in defining staff problem behaviors, scheduling meetings with the parties involved, and identifying issues for the team to address (Drinka &

Streim, 1994). In some cases the group may need to call in an outside consultant to address a dysfunctional group system.

7. The focus should be on what the staff has accomplished rather than on mistakes. Positive feedback must be provided when good care and successful approaches are observed and should not be reserved for annual evaluations.
8. Staff salary and benefits should be reviewed. Salaries should be competitive with other special care programs in the area, with pay raises based on performance. Program directors should participate in the evaluation of all staff members of the special care program team.
9. Flexibility and humor in providing care should be encouraged. This approach sets the tone for a more relaxed atmosphere that not only benefits staff but also results in less stress and fewer behavior problems among residents.
10. Certified nursing assistant support groups can be helpful in providing a safe environment in which to share both positive and negative caregiving feelings and experiences. For a support group to be effective, confidentiality must be ensured. The group's facilitator should be highly skilled in validating staff concerns and moving the groups from the sharing of feelings and problems toward empowerment, the development of coping skills, and problem resolution. If it is not possible to identify a facilitator, such as a social worker, psychologist, or other employee who possesses these skills and is not in the position of supervising special care program staff within the organization, it may be necessary to contract with a community mental health professional or employee assistance program.

Adequate Staff Training

For many dementia programs recruiting and retaining staff are probably the most persistent management problems. Because of the urgency involved in hiring staff, people who have little or no experience in working with residents with dementia are often selected to work in a special care program and given no more than a brief orientation session before starting their jobs. For the programs that do not provide ongoing training in the care of people with dementia a high staff turnover rate will eventually result in an untrained staff.

The following points can help ensure adequate staff training:

1. Ideally, staff should be trained before starting their assigned job. This eliminates having to take staff away from their work, which can cause problems with staffing and can add stress for the new employee. Because of frequent staff turnover, facilities must be prepared to offer dementia training on a continuing basis as part of new staff orientation. In addition to the initial training, periodic in-services that are related to the care of people with dementia should be provided.

2. Staff training should include information on the disease process, communication techniques, management of challenging behaviors, care strategies, working with families, and stress reduction techniques for staff. Training should include both classroom and supervised practice with residents. Although it is essential that staff providing direct care be trained in the care of people with dementia, it is also important to ensure that all facility employees receive some training. Because most employees, including housekeeping, dietary, business office, and reception personnel, have daily contact with residents with dementia and their families, they should possess basic knowledge about dementia and an understanding of the philosophy of the special care program as well as the ability to use communication techniques and approaches to managing difficult resident behavior. For additional information on staff training, see Chapter 2.
3. Bulletin boards should be displayed in staff areas because they are important communication and teaching tools that promote the flow of information to members of the special care program staff. Bulletin boards can be used to provide current information on dementia research, treatment, and care management; to reinforce care management strategies previously learned; and to announce upcoming training programs, in-services, and community workshops on dementia. Members of the special care program staff, as well as staff from other areas of the facility, should be encouraged to contribute items for the bulletin board.
4. All members of the special care program staff should be given the opportunity to attend in-services and workshops on dementia. If limited funding prevents a facility from sending a group of employees to a community education program, a few staff members can be allowed to go with the understanding that they will be expected to present the information to the rest of the staff. All members of the special care program should have the opportunity to attend at least one community workshop or seminar per year. For presentations that are particularly important to the special care staff, consider bringing the speaker to the facility to present the information to staff members.

ADMINISTRATIVE SUPPORT

Lack of administrative support for the special care program and staff was listed as the seventh most frequently reported problem among survey respondents (28%). A commitment to high-quality care is demonstrated by program administrators when the value system expresses respect for staff and residents. Failure by administrators to listen to and validate staff concerns as well as support the staff in stressful situations and praise them for their accomplishments will contribute to poor staff morale and retention. In some cases managers of other departments and programs are not involved closely enough in the special care program. This situation can result in the prevention of direct care staff from other departments who are involved in the care of the residents with dementia (e.g., dietary, housekeeping, therapy) from being able to carry out their tasks. Communication among staff levels and departments may also be impeded (Lawton, Van Haitsma, & Klapper, 1994). The need for creative approaches to and flexibility in completing work assignments may not be understood by management who are not aware of or do not agree with the philosophy of the special care program. For example, the dietary department may need to make adjustments in the serving of meals according to the residents' functional level and their ability to remain seated to finish the meal.

The following suggestions can be incorporated:

1. Mandatory training should be provided for all management staff in the philosophy and elements of the special care program.
2. Job descriptions that are specific to dementia care should be developed for all staff from other departments who are involved in the special care program. Job descriptions set guidelines for employee and departmental roles and responsibilities.
3. Administrators must support special care program coordinators in fostering a spirit of cooperation among departments.
4. Administrators should support their staff in the use of nontraditional approaches to dementia care and in the use of creative staffing.

ADMISSION CRITERIA

The use of inadequate admission criteria was identified as a problem in the operation of special care programs by 19% of survey respondents. Frequently, applicants for admission to special care programs have not been evaluated for dementia. Lack of information about the applicant can result in inappropriate placement in a special care program. Symptoms of cognitive impairment may in fact be caused by acute and chronic illnesses, sensory impairments, or depression and not by a dementing disease.

The following steps should be taken for proper placement of applicants:

1. The program's admission policy should require a comprehensive evaluation for dementia that provides the following information:
    - Results of diagnostic tests
    - Medical history
    - Behavior observations
    - Social history
    - Drug and alcohol use
    - Memory, language, motor, and personality functioning
2. The standards developed by the Joint Commission on Accreditation of Healthcare Organizations (1994) for special care programs should be used to develop or revise admission/discharge criteria.

3. Discharge criteria must be established for residents who are found to be inappropriately placed in the program or who cannot benefit from a special care program. Examples may include 1) residents with existing psychiatric disorders who cannot be managed in a special care program and who may be at risk of causing harm to other residents or to staff and 2) residents in an advanced state of a dementing disease who, because of their frailty, their inability to communicate, and their care needs (e.g., tube feeding, catheter, oxygen), may be vulnerable and at risk of harm by other more physically healthy residents with dementia. Catheter bags, intravenous setups, and oxygen masks often present attractive distractions to the confused resident who wanders into other residents' rooms. Whereas some facilities provide a separate section within a special care program for residents who are in advanced stages of dementia, others find it more feasible to transfer these residents to another area of the facility designed for residents who require a higher level of care.

Table 1.2 contains suggested program admission and discharge criteria.

ADDITIONAL CHALLENGES

In addition to the problems cited in the conference survey, several other issues present challenges in the provision of care to people with dementia.

Nutrition

Ensuring that residents with dementia receive adequate nutrition is a challenge throughout all stages of their illness. For residents in the early and middle stages of the disease, memory loss can disrupt familiar patterns of eating. Residents experiencing short-term memory loss may not remember their last meal and may insist that they have not eaten. Others who have a loss of appetite combined with disorientation to time will need to be cued or reminded to eat. Residents with dementia often refuse to sit and eat a complete meal, getting up to wander after a few bites. Residents who progress into a more advanced stage of dementia lose the ability to feed themselves and have difficulty swallowing their food.

The following approaches to help ensure good nutrition should be considered:

1. Create alternative eating arrangements with flexible serving times.
2. Have nutritional snacks available in the special care program at all times.
3. Provide finger foods for the wanderer that can be eaten while the resident moves about. Create a "wanderer's table" located apart from other residents' tables and assign a nursing assistant to supervise the table. Seat residents who tend to wander at this table and allow them to come and go.
4. Identify and make available residents' favorite foods. Solicit input from family members about residents' special preferences.

5. Try to redirect residents who insist that they have not been fed when in fact they have to an activity that will change their focus. If this does not work, provide them with a small snack.
6. Assign the same staff member to assist or feed the resident with dementia, whenever possible. Doing so allows that person to learn the most effective means of providing adequate food intake for that resident. A consistent approach by a familiar face helps to reduce mealtime stress for both staff and residents.
7. Reduce stimuli in the eating area by eliminating excessive noise such as music and staff chatter.

For additional suggestions in dealing with nutritional issues in dementia care, see the Supplemental Reading List at the back of the book.

Staff–Family Conflict

It is difficult for families to accept the cognitive and functional decline of a family member with dementia. Family members who are critical of the care provided by staff are often experiencing guilt and frustration associated with caregiving responsibilities and institutional placement as well as trying to deal with the impact of the resident's dementing illness on the disruption of family relationships and roles. In addition, the staff sees the family as a source of criticism regarding the resident's care, creating the potential for family and staff conflict over the resident's treatment plan (Maas et al., 1994).

The following suggestions may help in the effort to avoid or resolve conflict:

1. Develop programs and policies for the special care program to encourage the continued participation of family members in care planning and provision.
2. Orient families to the philosophy and policies of the special care program at the time of admission.
3. Include the family in care planning. The family is an important source of information about the resident's history, likes, and dislikes.
4. Establish a family council that addresses resident care issues and family–staff conflicts.
5. Organize a caregiver support group to provide peer support in dealing with feelings of guilt, frustration, and grief.
6. Arrange for the nursing facility ombudsman to meet with families when conflict cannot be resolved between families and staff.

Documentation

Chart documentation in a special care program presents an added burden to a staff already overwhelmed by the paperwork necessary to meet regulations and standards. An increasing amount of staff time is spent on special charting for problem behaviors, particularly when chemical and

Table 1.2. Guidelines for special care program admissions and discharges

Options for residents

- Residents are admitted who are in various stages of dementia and remain in the program until death (ambulatory residents are mixed with advanced stage residents).
- Residents are selected whose functional capabilities enable them to participate and benefit from therapeutic programs. Residents are discharged from the program when they are no longer able to participate in or benefit from the program.
- Residents are admitted who have a moderate level of functioning and are moved to a separate area within the unit for advanced-stage dementia.
- Residents on other floors who are exhibiting early signs of memory loss and other cognitive impairments and who have a diagnosis of dementia may participate in the daily program of activities in the special care program.

Admission criteria

- Confirmed dementia (other causes of condition such as delirium, other illness, sensory loss, or medication are ruled out)
- Stable medical condition
- Ability to participate in program activities
- Absence of behavior disorders that are beyond the program's care or safety capacity

Preadmission assessment

- Review of evaluation for dementia, which should include blood chemistry screening; neurology examination; mental status testing; psychosocial assessment; computed tomography scan, magnetic resonance imaging, electroencephalogram (as ordered by physician); and psychiatric and/or neuropsychological evaluation (when indicated)
- Evaluation of cognitive, physical, and social functioning within the preadmission environment
- Review of nursing notes if in a facility or hospital
- Psychosocial history
- Type and degree of family support, understanding, and acceptance of the disease process

Discharge criteria (dependent on resident population)

- An unstable or complex medical condition that requires acute or specialized care
- Functional status that is significantly reduced, resulting in total dependency in activities of daily living (e.g., eating, bathing, toileting) and high level of care required (e.g., feeding tube, oxygen)
- A behavioral problem that causes danger to self or others
- Resident cannot participate in or benefit from program activities because of one of the above situations or misdiagnosis or improvement in status

Discharge assessment

- Review any changes in residents' condition in care plan meeting.
- Reassess residents as their medical condition and functional status change.

physical restraints are used. Care plan documentation does not always address problems specific to dementia.

Consider the following suggestions to help reduce the burden of paperwork:

1. Use automated systems to reduce the amount of paperwork. Software has been developed to provide a comprehensive resident profile and assist with documentation in daily charting. The Veterans Affairs system has been working to create a database for some of their geriatric care programs to facilitate diagnosis, treatment planning, charting, research, and quality assurance (Department of Veterans Affairs, 1993).
2. Make care plan documentation specific in identifying approaches to care and behavior management. A quick-reference sheet that documents personal care needs, level of social and functional ability, and successful approaches to problem behaviors is helpful for all members of the special care program staff. This information-at-a-glance is particularly useful for new staff members.

CONCLUSIONS

A variety of experience in the planning and implementation of dementia-specific care is beginning to emerge. Whereas some approaches have been based on scientific theory and research, other methods have evolved from trial and error. Many pioneers in dementia care have faced the daily challenges of enhancing the quality of life for people with dementia without the benefit of research or guidelines to support their decisions. A systematic research agenda that examines the complexities of providing care to people with dementia was initiated by the National Institutes of Health (Cohen, 1994). It is hoped that through these studies and others, essential information and direction will soon be available to assist policymakers, government regulators, planners, and administrators in meeting the needs of people with dementia.

REFERENCES

Berg, L. (1984). Clinical dementia rating. *British Journal of Psychiatry, 145*, 339.

Berg, L. (1988). Clinical dementia rating. *Psychopharmacological Bulletin, 24*, 637–639.

The Brookdale Foundation. (1991). *How to start and manage a group activities and respite program for people with Alzheimer's disease and their families.* New York: Author.

Cohen, G.D. (1994). Toward new modes of dementia care. *Alzheimer's Disease and Associated Disorders, 8*(1), S2–S4.

Department of Veterans Affairs. (1993). *Survey of dementia services phase III: Dementia special care units.* Washington, DC: Office of Geriatrics and Extended Care, Veterans Health Administration.

Drinka, T.J.K., & Streim, J.E. (1994). Case studies from purgatory: Maladaptive behavior within geriatric health care teams. *Gerontologist, 34*(4), 541–547.

Hughes, C.P., Berg, L., Danziger, W.L., Cohen, L.A., & Martin, R.L. (1982). A new clinical scale for the staging of dementia. *British Journal of Psychiatry, 140,* 566–572.

Joint Commission on Accreditation of Healthcare Organizations. (1994). *Standards and survey protocol for dementia special care units.* Chicago: Author.

Kaplan, M. (1996). *Clinical practice with caregivers of dementia patients.* Washington, DC: Taylor & Francis.

Kaplan, M., & Parr, J. (1995). *Training teen volunteers in dementia care.* Paper presented at the Gerontological Society of America annual meeting, Los Angeles.

Kenshalo, D.R. (1977). Age changes in touch, vibration, temperature, kinesthesis, and pain sensitivity. In J.E. Birren & K.W. Schaie (Eds.), *Handbook of the psychology of aging* (pp. 562–579). New York: Van Nostrand.

Lawton, M.P., Van Haitsma, K., & Klapper, J. (1994). A balanced stimulation and retreat program for a special care dementia unit. *Alzheimer's Disease and Associated Disorders, 8*(1), S133–S138.

Maas, M.M., Buckwalter, K.C., Swanson, E., Specht, J., Tripp-Reimer, T., & Hardy, M. (1994). The caring partnership: Staff and families of persons institutionalized with Alzheimer's disease. *American Journal of Alzheimer's Care and Related Disorders and Research, 9*(6), 21–30.

Office of Technology Assessment. (1987, April). *Losing a million minds: Confronting the tragedy of Alzheimer's disease and other dementias* (Publication No. OTA-BA-323). Washington, DC: U.S. Government Printing Office.

Reisberg, P., Ferris, S.H., deLeon, M.J., & Crook, T. (1982). The global deterioration scale for assessment of primary degenerative dementia. *American Journal of Psychiatry, 139,* 1136–1139.

Smith, D.B. (1995). Staffing and managing special care units for Alzheimer's patients. *Geriatric Nursing, 16*(3), 124–127.

2

Training Staff to Work in Special Care

Mary Guerriero Austrom, Ph.D.

The single most important element in a good special care program is the staff. No unit, no matter how modern, efficient, well planned, and attractively decorated, can function well without carefully selected and trained staff members. Many administrators feel that money spent on training is not well spent. However, some administrators fail to take into account that money is lost in sick leave, high turnover rates, absenteeism, and issues related to job stress. Turnover rates for unlicensed staff in nursing facilities have been reported to range from 20% to 500% (Waxman, Carner, & Berkenstock, 1984). According to Waxman and coworkers, approximately 90% of the actual personal care in nursing facilities is provided by unlicensed staff. A review of the literature on nursing assistants working in nursing facilities showed turnover rates to range from 40% to 75% (Caudill & Patrick, 1989). These high turnover rates directly affect both the financial expenditures of the facility and the quantity and quality of care provided (Caudill & Patrick, 1989). Thus, addressing the training and support needs of nursing facility staff is of

This work was supported by the Indiana Alzheimer's Disease Center and the National Institutes on Aging Grant No. PHS P30 A610133-01.

critical importance to the success of long-term care facilities and special care programs alike.

Szwabo and Stein (1993) describe nursing facility work as both physically and emotionally demanding. In addition, many long-term care facility employees work for near-minimum wage and have only a high school education with limited opportunity for state-of-the-art training in long-term care approaches. These employees also have few options for career advancement or for peer collegial recognition (Helper, 1987; Lyons, Hammer, Johnson, & Silberman, 1987; Szwabo & Stein, 1993). Comprehensive staff training and continuing education and support could have an impact on staff morale, staff–resident interaction skills, and staff–residents' families relationships and could also benefit the long-term care facility, as measured in lowered levels of staff turnover, absenteeism, and job stress. This chapter describes a comprehensive staff training and support program that has been effective in several special care programs.

OVERVIEW OF THE TRAINING INTERVENTION PROGRAM

An educational intervention program was designed to meet the training needs of staff members of three special care programs in a large long-term care facility. The author developed the training program in conjunction with the assistant administrator of the facility and the directors of nursing and education, with the help of anonymous staff responses to a short survey about their own concerns about caring for residents with dementia (see the appendix at the end of this chapter). Researchers have found that adult learners should be involved in the process of diagnosing their training needs (Frazier & Sherlock, 1994; Knowles, 1969) and that this involvement keeps them interested in the educational process.

The overall goals of the training program were as follows:

1. Increase staff knowledge about Alzheimer's disease and related dementing disorders
2. Increase staff knowledge about resident management strategies and techniques
3. Increase the number of appropriate staff responses to noted resident incidents

In addition, the following objectives were set in place to meet the goals and evaluate the effectiveness of the program:

1. Increase staff knowledge about Alzheimer's disease and resident management issues through a variety of methods, including lectures, videotaped presentations, and case analyses
2. Audit resident charts pre- and post-training to evaluate application of learning
3. Evaluate staff knowledge using pre- and post-training tests
4. Increase staff morale through a supportive learning environment

The training program was delivered to staff members in 2-hour intervals every other week for 8 weeks. The author and colleagues have found that frequent short training sessions are more conducive to retention of new information than are longer sessions. By meeting every other week, the staff had the opportunity to implement new techniques and return with questions or comments. Sessions included the following:

- Overview of Alzheimer's disease
  - Basic diagnostic information
  - Early signs and symptoms
- Common problems associated with memory loss
  - Resident denies memory loss
  - Resident does not try to remember
  - Fluctuations in memory
  - Repetitive questions
  - Accusations
  - Lowered inhibitions

  This session included examples of typical interpretations of problem behaviors followed by more appropriate ways of interpreting the same behaviors. This exercise was particularly beneficial to staff members and helped them to attribute problem behaviors to the disease and not to the resident. A detailed description of this part of the training program can be found elsewhere in the chapter.
- Resident behavior: Appropriate versus inappropriate staff responses

  Examples of resident behavioral problems and staff responses to the problems were taken from audits of the residents' charts and used for discussing more appropriate ways of dealing with the problems.
- Communicating with the resident with Alzheimer's disease
  - Stages of decline in communication skills and how to help
  - Nonverbal communication
- Coping with challenging behaviors
  - Depression
  - Wandering
  - Catastrophic reactions
  - Hoarding
  - Suspicions and accusations
- Family members as allies
- A team approach to care

  It was important for both the staff and administration that the staff members learn to function as one team. One training session was devoted to discussing teamwork from a multidisciplinary perspective and ways to support one another in the special care program.

DATA COLLECTION

In order to measure the success of any training program, baseline measures must be obtained on which to make comparisons and draw conclusions about the effectiveness of training. However, it is not enough to provide an educational or training program and obtain a simple reaction-level evaluation of the program (i.e., did you like/dislike the program?). Reaction-level evaluations do not adequately assess transfer of learning, such as determining whether the participants learned anything or, more important, whether behavioral changes have taken place as the participants implement what they have learned in their work with residents with Alzheimer's disease. Therefore, multilevel evaluations, as proposed by Kirkpatrick (1967, 1976), were incorporated into this training program in order to examine different aspects of the value of the program. (*Note:* Staff members in two of the three special care programs were trained; the third group served as a control and the members were trained later. However, all three groups were evaluated.)

Alzheimer's Disease Awareness Questionnaires

All staff members (N = 18) were administered Alzheimer's disease awareness questionnaires (30 true/false items based on a training manual for nursing assistants by Helm & Weckstein [1991]) pre-training and 8 weeks post-training. These data provided a learning-level evaluation; that is, the data indicated whether the adult learners had absorbed and retained new information. In addition, reaction-level evaluations were obtained by a short program evaluation form designed for this study and administered to the staff at the end of the training program.

Evaluation of Staff–Resident Interaction

A total of 55 resident charts were audited before and after the training. The frequency and type of incidents reported by the staff were recorded, as well as the responses of the staff to the incidents. The information gathered from the audit of the charts was coded blindly and independently by the author and a nurse clinician. Behaviors were categorized by the author and a nurse clinician as follows:

- Expected behavior: Behavior that should not have been noted, such as wandering, having trouble remembering, and denying memory loss.
- Catastrophic reaction: All aggressive behavior toward others (e.g., staff, visitors, other residents) and any combination of the following symptoms with or without aggression—anxiety and agitation; emotional outburst; and paranoia, noncooperative behavior, and sexual incidents (Mace & Rabins, 1991).
- Agitation/anxiety/emotional outbursts: Behaviors that often accompany each other—resident unable to stop crying, wants to go home,

cannot find family members, paces, wrings hands, or yells or screams for no apparent reason, but is not physically aggressive.

- Paranoia and suspiciousness: Resident accuses others of stealing or being "out to get me" without symptoms associated with a catastrophic reaction.
- Noncooperative behavior: Resident will not bathe, eat, take medications, or change clothes without any sign of aggression or emotional agitation as described earlier.
- Bizarre behavior: Resident exhibits unusual behaviors such as eating soap, without anxiety or aggression.
- Inappropriate sexual behavior: Resident fondles self in public, grabs or fondles others, directs sexually offensive language toward others.

The responses of staff members to each recorded incident were also categorized independently and blindly by the author and a nurse clinician as follows:

- No response noted: Chart notes were left blank after an incident report.
- Appropriate response: Staff member intervened before the situation got out of hand by distracting or removing the resident; allowed the person to wander safely; consoled and comforted an agitated and emotionally distraught resident; showed compassion, empathy, and respect; and administered psychotropic medications in cases in which there was a clear history of repeated behavioral problems and in which environmental or behavioral interventions had not been effective.
- Inappropriate response: Trying to reason with the resident; expecting a rational explanation from the resident; using physical or chemical restraints when unnecessary (i.e., when the situation did not seem extreme or dangerous) or administering psychotropic drugs without documentation of a history of repeated problems or without documentation of behavioral and environmental modification attempts; and noting "will monitor situation" without any intervention or follow-up recorded. A reaction is inappropriate if it is not completed or if follow-up is insufficient.

The chart audits also provided information about the types of behavioral problems that were causing the most difficulty for staff members. It also became apparent which residents were the most challenging and where the staff lacked skills to deal effectively with the problem behaviors. The information taken from the charts provided the cases for training examples. Eight weeks after the last training session, the charts were reaudited. Behavioral-level evaluations of the program were obtained by examining resident charts and noting changes in the frequency of incident reports and types of staff reactions. It was possible to determine whether the staff had implemented what they learned and changed the way they responded to behavioral problems in residents.

RESULTS OF CHART AUDITS AND TRAINING PROGRAM

Alzheimer's Disease Awareness Questionnaires

Staff performance on the Alzheimer's disease awareness questionnaires increased after training for the staff of the two trained special care programs, whereas performance remained unchanged for the control group staff over the 8-week period. These results indicated that the staff members absorbed the information and retained it during the training period and at 8-week follow-up. In addition, all staff rated the program, materials, and the instructor highly, indicating a positive reaction-level evaluation.

Evaluation of Staff–Resident Interaction

At baseline, appropriate intervention was noted in 38.2% of the incidents recorded in the resident charts. At 8 weeks post-training, appropriate responses to incidents increased to 63.1%. These results strongly support the effectiveness of training and its impact on how the staff manages resident behaviors. It must be noted that the incidents did not stop; resident behavior was expected to remain consistent given a diagnosis of dementia.

At baseline, 29.1% of all reported incidents had been categorized as expected behaviors, events that should not have been noted in the charts as incidents. After training, in which a significant amount of time was spent with the staff discussing common problems associated with memory loss and behaviors that are common and expected with a diagnosis of Alzheimer's disease, the number of expected behaviors noted as incidents dropped to 10%. Although the study had been designed to keep staff members of one special care program untrained to serve as a control group, the number of appropriate interventions increased in all three programs. This result may have occurred because several of the trained staff members served as "floaters," staff members who worked in all three programs as needed. In addition, it was difficult to prevent staff members from discussing the training with their colleagues.

Many special care programs use floaters to cover for absent staff; therefore it is essential to train floaters and any staff who routinely work in the program along with the direct care staff. For example, housekeeping and dietary staff benefit from participating in several parts or all of the training program on dementia and common behavioral problems associated with memory loss. It is strongly recommended that all long-term care staff participate in a minimum of two in-services annually on dementia, its behavioral concomitants, and communication skills that are effective with people with dementia. It may be helpful to include a discussion of these issues as part of the routine orientation of all new staff.

MAJOR CONCLUSIONS OF TRAINING PROGRAM EVALUATION

The results of this study indicate the success of the training, but, more important, they emphasize the need for education in long-term care facilities. Staff members are not uncaring, but rather they are unprepared to deal with the special needs of residents with dementia. An added benefit of the program was the influence on the staff's perception of residents with Alzheimer's disease. Rather than viewing the residents as problematic, the staff learned to attribute the behavioral problems to the disease and not to hold the residents or themselves responsible for the difficulties. This in turn increased staff morale as staff began to feel more competent and confident dealing with the behavioral challenges posed by Alzheimer's disease.

As the training program progressed, a transition took place. Staff members began to support and provide information to one another. The trainer became a facilitator of discussion, and staff helped one another by sharing techniques they found useful in dealing with specific residents. This transition in the training process also marked the beginning of the team building process. Staff members began to understand the importance of working cohesively.

The training intervention program incorporated various methods to foster and apply learning, including case analyses of the staff's own residents, which made learning more meaningful. The frequent short training sessions are a departure from some training programs, which are often one-shot, intensive programs that do not have follow-up with the staff. A beneficial side effect of the author's program was the camaraderie experienced by the staff and the opportunity provided for them to voice concerns about their job, the residents, and organizational problems in a supportive environment. By the third training session, the atmosphere at the meetings changed from a formal classroom atmosphere to a support group atmosphere. As staff members began to trust the instructor and their colleagues and felt more confident about their resident management skills, they began to relax and enjoy the educational process. This camaraderie further encouraged and increased learning. Much has been written about offering support groups to staff members of special care programs, yet little empirical data exist about the effectiveness of such groups (Peppard, 1991). Although the study outlined in this chapter did not measure the effects of staff support per se, staff morale as evidenced by the instructor and measured by gratuitous self-reports increased tremendously.

GUIDELINES FOR DEVELOPING A TRAINING INTERVENTION PROGRAM

As the author has worked with various facilities and staff members since the mid-1980s, and developed numerous training programs for different types of facilities, several common guidelines or principles of successful training experiences have emerged, as follows. Try to incorporate some or all of these into your training early to ensure success.

1. Enlist staff members to help develop the program. Staff members will be more willing to engage in training sessions, participate more fully, and appreciate the value of training if they have been involved in the process from the beginning.
2. Discover what staff members know, what they do not know, and what they want to know. An effective way to uncover this information is to use an education and training survey such as the one in the Appendix.
3. Set clear goals and objectives. Setting clear goals and objectives will help define the length of the training program, frequency of meetings, and measurements of success.
4. Train, train, and train some more. Small doses of information can go a long way. Staff members will learn more if they have the opportunity to apply their newly acquired knowledge and skills and then return to the next training session with questions and concrete examples.
5. Do not reinvent the wheel; use existing training packages and handouts. Many special care program directors feel that they are not qualified to provide training because they do not know where to begin. However, there are many training programs on the market today that are excellent starting points for staff training. (Readers should refer to the supplemental reading and resources list at the back of the book for information on some training programs.) Incorporating examples from resident charts is also useful and do not require a large investment of time.
6. A training program is only as good as its trainer. If your facility does not have an experienced educator on staff, hire one. The training director should not only be knowledgeable about Alzheimer's disease and long-term care but must be an interesting, dynamic, and entertaining speaker. If the trainer does not possess these qualities, staff will lose interest and will not learn. Learning is also impeded if training is scheduled at shift changes.
7. Offer staff support. In developing the program, it quickly became apparent to the author that the staff members involved in the training program needed a safe place to voice concerns and frustrations related to the job or other, perhaps unrelated, concerns. Because working with residents with dementia is stressful, having the opportunity to unwind and discuss difficult issues is extremely valuable to staff members. The author recommends building a support group meeting time of an hour or an hour and a half into the staff's monthly schedule. Depending upon the cohesiveness of the staff, the group meeting can be directed by someone in the facility, such as the director of nursing,

a social services worker, or the director of the special care program. However, if tensions exist between the staff and supervisors, it is recommended that an outside facilitator be hired to help organize the group meetings. The author has found that it is often difficult to be both a supervisor and an objective listener.

8. Acknowledge and reward the efforts and accomplishments of the staff. Everyone appreciates and deserves a pat on the back. Recognize any special efforts made by staff members. Apply "The Golden Rule": Treat staff members as you would like to be treated. Extend respect and treat them with dignity. Thank them often for all they do. Acknowledge positive comments made about a staff member by a resident or a resident's family member. Reward perfect attendance or fewest absent or sick days. Hold a staff social; select an employee of the month; and publicize important events in staff members' lives, such as marriage and the birth of children. These activities help to build a team.

BARRIERS TO DEVELOPING AN EFFECTIVE TRAINING INTERVENTION PROGRAM

The barriers to developing an effective training intervention program are twofold, as follows:

1. Stressors that are beyond the ability of staff members to control. Training alone is inadequate if staff members face such stressors. For example, if the program is constantly short-staffed or if there is no safe place for residents to wander, the effects of training are easily undermined.
2. The administration of the long-term care facility does not demonstrate a commitment to the special needs of residents with Alzheimer's disease and their families, or a commitment to the training program. Making these commitments is essential to the success of the training program. Staff members should be compensated for training time, and their time spent in training should be recorded in their employment histories.

ELEMENTS OF A SUCCESSFUL TRAINING PROGRAM

Responding to Common Problems

An important key for staff in meeting the challenges of caring for residents with Alzheimer's disease is understanding some of the common behavioral manifestations of memory loss. The most striking discovery made about the chart audits was the staff's comments about difficult incidents. As the following examples from the chart audit indicate, staff members lacked basic information about Alzheimer's disease and other dementing disorders and knowledge about how to manage or respond to the behavioral manifestations of the disease. Most staff members are happy to have the opportunity for continuing education. The following are portions of the author's training program that staff members have found particularly beneficial.

Resident Behavior

A resident refused her medication, became agitated, and began yelling, "No! No!"

Staff Reaction

I could not reason with the resident.

Resident Behavior

A resident accused several other residents of taking her sweater and told everyone that they were thieves.

Staff Reaction

The staff member tried to tell her that each resident has his or her own clothes and that those clothes do not belong to her. The resident would not listen.

Resident Behavior

A resident was in the hallway with his coat on. A staff member asked him where he was going. The resident ignored the question and left the building.

Staff Reaction

The staff member followed the resident and made continued efforts to ask him where he was going. The resident would not say why he left the unit and would not talk about what was on his mind.

One of the most rewarding parts of the training program for trainers and learners alike is teaching the staff some basic behavior management techniques and working through examples from their own programs. Rather than try to modify the resident's behaviors by reasoning and rationalizing, staff members learned that it is their responsibility to adapt their own behavior and learn to respond to residents in new ways. It is essential for staff to remember that the resident is not willfully or purposefully "misbehaving."

If the staff can understand and learn to accept the changes and behaviors described rather than attempt to modify resident behavior, a major hurdle to effective care has been crossed. Discussing these common problems early in the training program helps to shift the emphasis away from "problem residents" to problems caused by the disease. Once caregivers accept the fact that the residents' actions or words are unintentional and redefine the problem behaviors as a consequence of the disease, the challenges of care are seen in a different light and they can "forgive" the resident and themselves for some of the difficulties. The following paragraphs provide examples of some common misinterpretations of resident behavior followed by appropriate ways of interpreting the behavior.

Resident denies the memory loss. Often, caregivers are frustrated when residents simply will not admit they are having trouble remembering. It is important for the staff to understand that residents have suffered memory loss and are unable to remember. For the resident, an appropriate and adaptive short-term emotional response is denial. Denial is a way of protecting one's sense of self by believing "This is not happening to me," or "I am not having this trouble." The resident may try to cover up the memory loss or direct frustration at the caregiver by becoming angry when confronted with reality. Protracted denial is maladaptive because it often interferes with important long-range planning.

Once long-range legal and financial issues are addressed, it is much more humane to allow residents their own reality rather than force them to accept the truth. As the dementing disease progresses and short-term memory continues to fade, many residents live in the past because long-term memory remains intact. It is better for these residents to be allowed to live with the things that are the most comforting. Many residents decline to the point that they no longer recognize themselves in a mirror, yet they are able to recognize photographs of their wedding or school graduation.

Staff should encourage family members to bring in photographs of the resident when he or she was younger. Working closely with family caregivers to learn a little about the resident's past can help establish a relationship with both the resident and the family. Another way to help preserve the resident's identity for staff members and visitors is to place a photograph of the resident and a brief biography of his or her life on the door to his or her room. This information also provides visitors with ideas for conversation, which can be difficult at times.

Resident does not try to remember. A major problem associated with Alzheimer's disease is lack of attention span, yet caregivers often feel that the resident is simply being lazy. It seems to the caregiver that residents could remember if they would try harder and pay attention. In the earliest stages of the disease, stimulating the resident's memory may be helpful; for example, keep a calendar or a list of medications that must be taken. However, the caregiver should not try to perform activities designed to stimulate cognitive functioning because this frustrates the resident even more. Do not force the resident to remember or insist that he or she try harder. Instead offer him or her the information or ask questions about what he or she is trying to accomplish. Compensate for the resident's cognitive functioning losses.

Resident's memory fluctuates. Just as we all have our good days and bad days, so does the person with Alzheimer's disease. His or her mood and memory may fluctuate as a result of exercise, nutrition, hydration, side effects of medication, and presence or absence of pain. When these fluctuations occur, they tend to reinforce the misconception that the resident does not try to remember or only remembers what he or she wants to remember. However, fluctuations in memory and cognitive skills are quite normal. Take advantage of the good days by encouraging walks, participation in activities, and outings. Accept the bad days and help the resident cope with ups and downs by remaining supportive and uncritical of his or her remaining abilities.

Resident asks repetitive questions. Caregivers often feel the resident is asking repetitive questions to annoy them; it seems that surely he or she can control the behavior, given that the question has been answered 15 times in 10 minutes. Caregivers must keep in mind that the person cannot remember having asked the question 15 times already. The resident no longer has the skills to gain attention appropriately and may actually be attempting to communicate pain, fear, or some other concern. It is important to pay attention to the resident's nonverbal cues in order to decipher an underlying problem.

If the resident appears calm and is not in physical or psychological pain, staff should try distracting him or her with a walk (outside if the weather permits), a favorite snack, or an activity. However, if the person is behaving in an anxious or agitated manner, he or she may be in some physical or emotional pain. Staff members should try to calm the person, move him or her to a quiet area, check for obvious sources of pain, and remain calm and comforting.

Resident makes accusations. A resident may constantly accuse caregivers or others of stealing his or her possessions, which leaves caregivers frustrated or angry. Accusing others is one way for the person to save face and cope with the insecurity caused by being unable to remember where he or she has put things. Staff members should respond to the accusations calmly, suggest that perhaps the item was misplaced, and help look for it. If this behavior is displayed often, the caregiver may discover that the person has a favorite hiding place. If the item cannot be found easily, distract the resident with an activity, a snack, or an outing. If the "lost" item is important, staff should suggest to the family that they might bring in an extra. Staff should always try to remain calm and reassuring.

Resident has lowered inhibitions. A previously demure resident may begin behaving in sexually inappropriate ways. These behaviors are not indicative of premorbid personality traits but are additional symptoms of the dementing disease. Damage to certain areas of the brain as a result of Alzheimer's disease often leads to a loss of impulse control. The person simply cannot help acting as he or she does. Defining the problem as a function of the disease helps caregivers (staff and family members alike) to cope with the behaviors more effectively.

Residents' rights must be protected; but if the inappropriate behavior is upsetting others, the caregiver should calmly distract the resident and remove him or her from the area. If one resident is annoying another, they should be separated calmly and gently. Staff must not overreact. Residents can sense their caregiver's emotional state from behaviors, even if they no longer comprehend the spoken word. Residents can also feel shame, disgrace, and pain, even if they cannot communicate. Therefore, it is important that these situations be handled with sensitivity.

When a person has dementia, it does not mean that he or she no longer needs or desires human contact. On the contrary, a warm hug or soft touch may be what the person needs but can no longer ask for. Large stuffed animals or pets may fill a need for comfort. Do not overlook the possibility that an underlying physical cause or side effects of medication could be responsible for the inappropriate sexual behavior. Talk to the resident's physician.

Resident wanders. All behavior has a purpose, even if a person does not understand its meaning. For example, residents with Alzheimer's disease may wander because they are looking for something. They often search for something comforting, such as a childhood home or their mother. A resident may begin to wander in the late afternoon because for 35 years, late afternoon is when he or she went home from work. The need to leave the unit and go home is so strong and the pattern so ingrained that many residents without dementia also report a similar sense of restlessness in the late afternoon. A resident may wander because he or she is in pain and can no longer communicate that pain. It is up to the staff member to determine the underlying cause of the behavior. Although the problem-solving process may be time consuming initially, the benefits to the resident far outweigh the commitment of time. Finding adequate solutions to the problem of wandering, for example, is far more humane than chemical or physical restraints and preserves the resident's dignity.

Understanding and Coping with Losses in Communication

A fundamental problem in working with residents with Alzheimer's disease and other dementing illnesses appears to be difficulty in communicating. Because of this barrier, staff members report greater difficulty in resident management. Simply because a resident can no longer communicate verbally, however, does not mean that he or she is not trying to communicate. One of the greatest human needs is to be understood (Covey, 1989). Imagine, therefore, the psychological distress a person must feel when this is no longer possible via the usual methods. Residents may use other means to communicate, and it falls to the caregiver to decipher that meaning. A key issue for staff members to bear in mind is that these residents can no longer function rationally; therefore, they cannot change their behavior. Staff members still have rational control over their environment; therefore, they can change and adapt their behavior in order to help the person with Alzheimer's disease.

Communication skills deteriorate progressively in dementing illnesses. The following is a description of the most common communication difficulties experienced by these residents and ways in which caregivers can help. In the earliest stages of the disease, residents may have occasional difficulty finding words and remembering names of familiar objects or people, and they may substitute words that sound similar or have similar meanings. It is usually less frustrating for the residents to be given the correct word. However, if supplying the word is upsetting to residents, do not supply the word. When the word they are searching for is unclear, ask residents to show or describe what they mean, if possible.

As the disease progresses, the residents have greater difficulty communicating thoughts and may be able to say only a few words. Residents may ramble by stringing together commonly used phrases. The sentence may seem to make sense, but actually it does not. When these types of communication problems occur, the caregiver can try to guess what the resident wants to say. Caregivers should ask residents if they are guessing correctly; guessing incorrectly may confuse the resident further. They should respond to residents' feelings and be alert to nonverbal cues. When words no longer make sense, they should consider residents' emotional state and feelings. People with Alzheimer's disease retain the capacity to feel and experience emotions throughout the course of the illness.

In late-stage Alzheimer's disease, residents may remember only a few key words, may repeat phrases over and over, may cry out intermittently, and may mumble unintelligible phrases; eventually they may not speak at all. If a resident can still shake his or her head, the caregiver should ask simple questions about his or her needs. A regular routine of checking the resident's comfort should be established. The caregiver should ensure that the resident's clothing is comfortable, that the room is warm, that there are no sores or rashes on the skin, and that regular feeding and toileting procedures are established.

Coping with Family Members

Spouses usually seek long-term care when their mate can no longer be managed at home, often when the caregiver's health and physical resources fail. Adult child caregivers often have different motivations for placing a parent with Alzheimer's disease in a long-term care facility. As a result of the various demands on their time from families, careers, and civic responsibilities, adult children have been appropriately referred to as the "sandwich generation" (Brody, 1981). Often, they see long-term care as a solution to one of their problems. Although they may not visit as often as spouse caregivers or may live far away, their anger and guilt is often similar to that experienced by spouse caregivers.

Family caregivers often have a difficult time relinquishing control over their loved one's care, and their guilt is often expressed as anger toward the staff and the facility (Guerriero Austrom & Hendrie, 1990). Too often residents with "difficult" family members suffer the consequences. Staff members spend less time with the resident, set up barriers to effective communication, and avoid the family caregivers in order to protect themselves from further attack. If staff members can understand and appreciate the true cause of a family's anger, they can work to diffuse the anger and cultivate a collaborative relationship so that both parties "win" and the person receives optimal care.

Family members often express their concerns and fears as hostility toward the staff. The following lists fears and concerns commonly expressed by families and ways in which caregivers can help. By employing some of the following strategies to diffuse the anger, special care program staff and family members can become partners in the resident's care.

No one can care for my loved one like I can. No institution can provide 24-hour care like the family member, but that fact does not mean that care will be poor, only different. It is important for staff to acknowledge the family's fears and concerns, empathize with them, and respect their anxieties. It is important for staff members to listen with their hearts. The caregiver should ask him- or herself, How would I feel if it were my parent, spouse, or sibling who was being placed in a long-term care facility? The reality is that most of us will face a similar decision one day. Although staff are often busy with numerous residents, they should keep in mind that for each family this experience with long-term care is its only experience with this care and everything is new and confusing. Staff members need to be considerate of family feelings.

I am no longer an important part of my loved one's care. Staff should acknowledge the tremendous job family members have done so far and emphasize that their involvement in the resident's care has not ended. The family's help in providing the best care possible should be requested. With direction, encouragement, and appreciation, families can ease the staff's burden. The family should be prepared as to what to expect by explaining what the resident's daily routine will be and that the resident may become more disoriented at first. Staff should keep the family involved. Although this may be more time consuming initially, their involvement provides long-term benefits.

For many caregivers, especially spouses, caregiving was their primary role. Many caregivers had reduced or given up their jobs outside the home to care for their loved one. Thus, once the person is no longer at home, many family caregivers can become depressed. They are not only losing a loved one but also a sense of purpose in their lives. Family members may also feel guilty at having had to seek long-term care. They may be breaking a promise to a loved one who in the past may have asked not to be placed in a nursing facility. Family members may not be able to understand these feelings in themselves. Staff should be patient, supportive, and understanding of their losses. The first parting after the loved one has been admitted is often unbearable for family members. One family caregiver remembers fondly the staff member who called her at home the first evening after she had placed her mother in a special care program and told her how much fun her mother was having at a social event. This one small, thoughtful gesture was extremely comforting to a distraught daughter.

There is no privacy; other residents are always wandering in and out of the room. Family members should be made aware that most residents wander, and that it does not bother most of the other residents. If a family's loved one is agitated by this behavior, staff should try to respect the wishes for privacy whenever possible and apologize when necessary.

Staff do not spend enough time helping with meals. It always took me 2 hours to feed him or her. Staff should reassure the family that they are doing their best with the resident's feeding routine. The family's help at mealtime should be enlisted. Staff should ask what are the resident's favorite finger foods and arrange for them to be prepared. Field trips and outings should be arranged around mealtimes. Residents should be allowed to eat when they are hungry.

Personal belongings are always getting lost. Staff should encourage family members to remove valuables from the resident's room and to provide the resident with easy-care, loose-fitting clothing. Family complaints should always receive responses and staff should strive to avoid the problems that caused the complaint in the future. All staff members should be informed about a family's concerns so that the resident's care is consistent.

Staff are too busy to deal with us. An insightful and empathic staff member learned the interesting concept of the emotional bank account early in her career. (The concept is that if a person makes an emotional deposit, he or she has a balance from which to draw; if too much is withdrawn before a deposit is made, the person is operating in a deficit economy.) She reported how a family member of one of the residents under her care came to her extremely angry that the resident did not have her dentures and demanded to know where they were and how such a thing could happen. Rather than respond defensively with her own frustration and exasperation, the staff member dropped everything and conducted a thorough search of the resident's room, the special care program, and finally the kitchen until the dentures were found. Of course, the staff member was 2 hours behind in her charting, but she was miles ahead in her relationship with the family. She reported how appreciative and cooperative the family member became, how the anger and frustration dissipated, and how the family member now always has a warm smile for her.

In their pain families often look for things on which to focus their anger, such as missing dentures or misplaced articles of clothing. If staff can find the patience to listen and respond to the request, the rewards can be tremendous.

CONCLUSIONS

Caring for people with Alzheimer's disease is challenging. It is not difficult to understand why special care program staff become frustrated. However, by learning about the effects of the disease on the personality, staff members can become more understanding about the resident's behaviors and will be receptive to employing diverse management techniques. Through education, training, and ongoing support, staff members can become a cohesive team and partners with family members in helping to care for and preserve the dignity of the person with Alzheimer's disease.

REFERENCES

Brody, E.M. (1981). "Women in the middle" and family help to older people. *Gerontologist, 21,* 471–480.

Caudill, M., & Patrick, M. (1989). Nursing assistant turnover in nursing homes and need satisfaction. *Journal of Gerontological Nursing, 15*(6), 24–30.

Covey, S.R. (1989). *The seven habits of highly effective people.* New York: Fireside Books.

Frazier, C., & Sherlock, L. (1994). Staffing patterns and training for competent dementia care. In M.K. Aronson (Ed.), *Reshaping dementia care: Practice and policy in long-term care.* Thousand Oaks, CA: Sage Publications.

Guerriero Austrom, M., & Hendrie, H.C. (1990). Death of the personality: The grief response of the Alzheimer's disease family caregiver. *American Journal of Alzheimer's Care and Related Disorder and Research, 5*(2), 16–27.

Helm, B.J., & Wekstein, D.R. (1991). *For those who take care: An Alzheimer's disease training program for nursing assistants.* Lexington: Alzheimer's Disease Research Center, Sanders-Brown Center on Aging, University of Kentucky.

Helper, S. (1987). Assessing training needs of nursing home personnel. *Journal of Gerontological Social Work, 11,* 71–79.

Kirkpatrick, D.L. (1967). Evaluation of training. In R.L. Craig & L.R. Bittel (Eds.), *Training and development handbook* (pp. 87–112). New York: McGraw-Hill.

Kirkpatrick, D.L. (1976). Evaluation of training. In R.L. Craig (Ed.), *Training and development handbook: A guide to human resource development* (pp. 18-1–18-27). New York: McGraw-Hill.

Knowles, M. (1969). *Higher adult education in the United States: The current picture, trend, and issues.* Washington, DC: American Council on Education.

Lyons, J.S., Hammer, J.S., Johnson, N., & Silberman, M. (1987). Unit specific variation in occupational stress across a general hospital. *General Hospital Psychiatry, 9,* 435–438.

Mace, N.L., & Rabins, P.V. (1991). *The 36-hour day: A family guide to caring for persons with Alzheimer's disease, related dementing illness and memory loss in later life* (Rev. ed.). Baltimore: The Johns Hopkins University Press.

Peppard, N.R. (1991). *Special needs dementia units. Design, development and operations.* New York: Springer Publishing.

Szwabo, P.A., & Stein, A.L. (1993). Professional caregiver stress in long term care. In P.A. Szwabo & G.T. Grossberg (Eds.), *Problem behaviors in long-term care. Recognition, diagnosis, and treatment.* New York: Springer Publishing.

Waxman, H.M., Carner, E.A., & Berkenstock, G. (1984). Job turnover and job satisfaction among nursing home aides. *Gerontologist, 24*(5), 503–509.

APPENDIX

Education and Training Survey

In order to develop additional training in the area of dementia, Alzheimer's disease, resident care, and family caregiver issues, please answer the following questions.

1. What are the three most challenging or difficult issues you face when caring for residents with dementia?

   a.

   b.

   c.

2. If you have received previous training in this area or have attended workshops on Alzheimer's disease, what did you find most helpful about the training?

3. What did you find the least helpful about previous training programs?

4. Please check each topic that interests you:

   _____ Communicating with the person with Alzheimer's disease
   _____ Depression in the person with Alzheimer's disease
   _____ Behavioral management issues
   _____ Sexuality and the person with Alzheimer's disease
   _____ Managing staff stress
   _____ Understanding the family caregiver

5. What other information about Alzheimer's disease would you like to know more about?

3

Programming and Activities

Sylvia Nissenboim, A.C.S.W.

Many good years may await people who have received a diagnosis of Alzheimer's disease. There is, in fact, "life after diagnosis," an expression coined by Dr. Burton Reifler, Program Director of the Robert Wood Johnson's Partners in Caregiving Program. His words address the vital, positive approach to dealing with this disease.

Alzheimer's disease is a progressive disease that slowly destroys the independence, skills, memories, and knowledge acquired over a person's lifetime. On the average, between 7 and 12 years may pass between diagnosis and the person's death. The time at which a person receives the diagnosis may be the most critical time at which to focus on an individual's strengths and abilities. Faculties that will remain intact for many years should be capitalized upon. Newly diagnosed older adults must acknowledge the possibilities in the years ahead, during which they will still be able to participate in life's experiences.

Services and supports for people with dementia and their families are expanding along a continuum of care. From modified independent living to supervised work settings to adult day services and eventually to special care programs, programming along the continuum of care can help improve the quality of life for many years. Family members and professionals alike can design interventions to help people with Alzheimer's disease or related dementias maintain the courage to stay active and involved despite the deterioration associated with the disease. The Positive Interactions Program concentrates on the early, middle, and late stages of the disease from the person's perspective (Nissenboim & Vroman, 1995). Additionally, support groups, educational programs, and respite care programs are available. Only since the mid-1980s have support groups for cognitively impaired people been offered regularly in some areas.

People newly diagnosed with Alzheimer's disease have issues that must be confronted before they are ready for a higher level of acceptance. They must grieve, mourn, and come to terms with the inevitability of their loss of independence. They must learn how to accept help from loved ones when it is needed and not before. Otherwise, they will be abandoning their potential to retain skills and may exacerbate their disability. Additionally, they must realize that they still have a wealth of coping strategies that have been acquired throughout their lives, which they may continue to utilize. Coping styles and strategies are extremely important tools in the earliest stages of Alzheimer's disease. Many newly diagnosed people suffer from depression. They should be reassured that they are prepared to meet the future with their greatest resources—their emotional and physical health.

Geriatric assessment services help families and individuals to understand the whole picture and provide appropriate information and resource referrals. As the dementia progresses, adult day services programs and in-home services are extremely beneficial in order to maintain a stimulating and supervised environment. The key is to help maintain the person's involvement with relationships and surroundings, promoting independence and a healthy self-image. This is critical in order to meet the goal of reducing the effects of isolation and subsequent withdrawal from stimulating environments.

People in the early stages of Alzheimer's disease may participate in supervised work programs. These programs run similar to an office, in which people complete jobs that have been contracted from outside agencies. The objective of this program is to provide meaningful, success-oriented tasks that will engender pride in new work endeavors. Once a person is no longer able to perform the job-related tasks, he or she is more appropriately served by adult day services, where increased structure and supervision are provided.

THE POSITIVE INTERACTIONS PROGRAM

The person with cognitive impairment has lost the ability to understand and to be understood. Positive interactions offer the person the potential for successful opportunities and for development of a bond between the person and the caregiver.

The Positive Interactions Program (Nissenboim & Vroman, 1995) is designed to provide structured time within a hazy world. The program focuses attention on the different areas of strength to be found within the stages of Alzheimer's disease, and is a successful approach to activity development for older adults with cognitive impairment. It can also be a teaching model for caregivers to help them organize their days, enhance the time spent with clients, and decrease their frustration level as well as that of clients.

All caregivers must learn how to continue living with their failing, frustrated, frightened, and sometimes frightening parent, spouse, or client. This program helps caregivers to create favorable conditions for their relationships with the person with cognitive impairment, to become excited over the recognition of hidden abilities, and to understand that there can and will be moments of shared enjoyment and pleasure. In this program trained professionals enable clients' families to take a step back from caregiving. Family members can spend leisure time with their loved one, engaged in planned tasks that encourage the person with cognitive impairment in a sense of success and the family members in their ability to create a safe and rewarding environment.

Objectives of the Program

Too frequently, caregivers lose sight of the long-term goals that will support the person with cognitive impairment in his or her attempts to participate; short-term activities are mistakenly seen as the main objective. To encourage people with cognitive impairment, caregivers must focus on their involvement and satisfaction, not on the task or activity. The Positive Interactions Program stresses the use of activities as the tools for achieving person-oriented objectives.

The following guidelines should be followed in every interaction:

- Provide opportunities for success.
- Provide opportunities for quality interactions.
- Accept the person at his or her functional level.

Although many professional duties focus on performing tasks for the person with cognitive impairment, every professional should set aside time for "doing with" rather than "doing for" the person. The program focuses on interactions between two people. Caregivers should make statements that reflect their own pleasure and involvement in these interactions, which communicates to the person with cognitive impairment that the caregiver is also a receiver. The caregiver should talk about him- or herself. It is extremely important to support the sense of giving and receiving of the person with dementia. Most of the time, he or she is placed in a position of receiving. In order to achieve a better sense of balance, the person is credited for contributing to every interaction.

Considerations for the Caregiver

The Positive Interactions Program is well suited to both adult day services and long-term care facilities, providing activities, scheduling, and an approach that meets the facility's objective of caring for clients or residents along the prescribed "Quality of Care" guidelines of the Omnibus Budget Reconciliation Act of 1987 regulations. The program may be incorporated as the style of staff–client/resident interaction or as a regularly scheduled activity.

Adding the responsibilities associated with a new program may appear overwhelming, but administrators should realize that the staff burnout rate is usually highest when time is not structured for older adults with cognitive impairment. Lack of an organized activity plan can accentuate agitation, wandering, perseveration (repetition of something beyond a desired point), and emotional upset. When focused tasks are organized throughout the day, both caregivers and clients/residents feel a greater sense of stability.

A common and often unconscious response among family members is to treat their loved one as a patient or a child. Family members can be trained to rediscover positive ways to spend time with their loved one. Family members do not benefit from an around-the-clock caregiver–care receiver relationship; this relationship encourages the person to begin to feel more dependent than is necessary. Family relationships must be maintained as long as possible. Husband–wife, parent–child, sibling–sibling, and professional–client/resident relationships all have mutually satisfying aspects that can be rediscovered or reinvented. A husband and wife may find new ways of being intimate with each other as the disease progresses.

The person with Alzheimer's disease can be encouraged to rediscover ways to extend care to the caregiver. Creating opportunities for reciprocity in a very unbalanced situation can bridge gaps. Caregivers also need attention, and individuals with impairments need to be permitted to help out.

DESIGNING AN ACTIVITY PLAN

A wide selection of activities is crucial to the success of a program. Repeating the same activity too frequently may raise responses from the older adult such as "We just did that," or "This again?" The greater the variety of activities, the greater the chances of providing positive experiences.

Each activity described in the following sections is designed to be flexible in degree of complexity, allowing for adjustments in design. This flexibility helps the client/resident to achieve success and enjoyment within his or her current abilities.

A critical variable to be considered is the amount of assistance required. The activity can remain the same for an individual, but the degree of assistance he or she needs increases as the disease progresses. Verbal encouragement may be all that is needed in Stage 1 of dementia. However, as the disease progresses and the person appears frustrated with the activity, adjustments can be made. Assistance can range from verbal encouragement to demonstration to hand-in-hand assistance.

In designing an activity plan, one should give equal consideration to the factors of preference, ability, degree of assistance required, and degree of assistance available. Because these factors are unique to the individual and the evaluation of each varies among facilities, the appropriateness of the activity should be determined according to the Clinical Dementia Rating scale (Table 3.1). The Clinical Dementia Rating has been used in the Memory and Aging Project at Washington University–St. Louis since 1977. Its use in assessing the natural history of senile dementia of the Alzheimer's type has proved useful as a longitudinal measure of the course of the disease (Miller, 1988). This scale has wide acceptance for determining the stages of Alzheimer's disease and can be easily applied to measuring abilities (Morris, 1993). The activities described in the Positive Interactions Program are coded as to their appropriateness to each stage, as outlined in the Clinical Dementia Rating scale.

INTRODUCING ACTIVITIES

The following are some general guidelines for introducing an activity to a person with dementia.

Familiarize. Allow the person to handle the activity items. A general description may be provided. Give the person time to focus on, hear, and/or feel each object.

Name. Naming provides an auditory cue. Focus on one item, name it, and then move on to another one or two items. Speak slowly, and encourage participation by providing the person with time to name another person or an object. Never require the naming of an object or person, no matter how familiar. Anything that feels like testing will be frightening and frustrating. If the person with dementia names an object or person, always express pleasure. Reward any participation by a touch or a response such as "That's great!"

Many times, a person with dementia will supply an inappropriate or incorrect answer. In such cases gently try to get the person back on track. If the person stays with this focus, he or she may be trying to communicate something else. Follow his or her lead.

Demonstrate. Demonstrating provides visual and tactile information. If the activity has a process, demonstrate the steps necessary to perform it, preferably hand-in-hand with the person with dementia. This assistance encourages active participation from the person. Proceed at the individual's own speed and presume nothing. More than two or three steps might be too complex for the person. The facilitator's voice, tone, and descriptions should be kept calm, even, and simple.

Encourage and reward. The disorientation and subsequent frustration felt by the older adult with cognitive impairment in attempting to understand

Table 3.1. Clinical Dementia Rating

	Impairment				
	None 0	Questionable 0.5	Mild 1	Moderate 2	Severe 3
Memory	No memory loss or inconsistent slight forgetfulness	Consistent slight forgetfulness; partial recollection of events; "benign" forgetfulness	Moderate memory loss; more marked for recent events; defect interferes with everyday activities	Severe memory loss; only highly learned material retained; new material rapidly lost	Severe memory loss; only fragments remain
Orientation	Fully oriented	Fully oriented except for slight difficulty with time relationships	Moderate difficulty with time relationships; oriented for place at examination; may have geographic disorientation elsewhere	Severe difficulty with time relationships; usually disoriented to time, often to place	Oriented to person only
Judgment and problem solving	Solves everyday problems and handles business and financial affairs well; judgment good in relation to past performance	Slight impairment in solving problems, similarities, and differences	Moderate difficulty in handling problems, similarities, and differences; social judgment usually maintained	Severely impaired in handling problems, similarities, and differences; social judgment usually impaired	Unable to make judgments or solve problems

Community affairs	Independent function at usual level in job, shopping, and volunteer and social groups	Slight impairment in activities	Unable to function independently at these activities, although person may still be engaged in some; appears normal to casual inspection	No pretense of independent function outside home; appears well enough to be taken to outside functions	No pretense of independent function outside home; appears too ill to be taken to outside functions
Home and hobbies	Life at home, hobbies, and intellectual interests well maintained	Life at home, hobbies, and intellectual interests slightly impaired	Mild but definite impairment of function at home; more difficult chores abandoned; more complicated hobbies and interests abandoned	Only simple chores preserved; very restricted interests, poorly maintained	No significant function in home
Personal care	Fully capable of self-care	Fully capable of self-care	Needs prompting	Requires assistance in dressing, hygiene, retaining personal effects	Requires much help with personal care; frequent incontinence

Note: Score only as decline from previous usual level due to cognitive loss, not impairment due to other factors.

Adapted with permission from Morris, J. (1993, November). *Neurology, 43*(11), 2413.

is difficult to describe. To avoid feelings of inadequacy and intimidation, the person desperately needs honest praise and encouragement to continue in the effort to achieve. If humiliated or ignored, the person probably will not want to try to understand.

Rewarding participation provides emotional encouragement. Give a reward for every accomplishment. For the more distracted individual, completing a task is remarkable, and so is attending to an activity. People with dementia should never be spoken to as if they were children or patronized with empty rewards. The facilitator should emphasize his or her desire to spend this time together with the person and should show that it is also meaningful and enjoyable for him or her. A successful interaction should exhibit a sense of beginning, middle, and end: "You seemed to enjoy looking at those pictures. I enjoyed myself, too. Now let's get lunch ready."

ACTIVITY CATEGORIES

The objectives of the Positive Interactions Program are met by interactions between the caregiver and the person with cognitive impairment using a variety of activities, which may be grouped into the categories of sensory-focused tasks, activities of daily living (ADLs), and physical activities. Each activity category focuses upon different skills, all with opportunities for success.

The first category of activity involves the five senses: vision, smell, touch, hearing, and taste. Sensory-focused tasks are successful with people with dementia because they draw upon skills that may not be impaired to the same degree as is language. Many new opportunities may still be available, because a person's abilities are often inappropriately assessed based on language ability, which deteriorates early in dementia. With these tasks, the person with impairment actively uses the senses to identify, discriminate between, or be creative with the objects presented. Activities should include all of the sensory modes before ruling any of them to be inappropriate, because abilities that involve the senses are not apparent unless demonstrated and evaluated.

ADLs encompass household, outdoor, and personal care tasks. In an adult day services or long-term care facility, many facets of routine tasks may become part of a daily activity schedule. Through participation, the person with cognitive impairment may gain the benefits of success and feel useful.

Physical activities are excellent additions to an activity schedule. They burn off excess energy and provide stimulation. Planned physical activities can reduce the agitation that may lead to the wandering and excessive pacing that is typical in dementia.

Examples of activities in the Positive Interactions Program are included in the appendix to this chapter.

ACTIVITIES FOR STAGE 1 OF DEMENTIA

Most individuals in Stage 1 of dementia will still be under the care of an attending physician rather than in an adult day services program or a long-term care facility. Therefore, the level of difficulty of activities should focus on the latter period of this stage.

The person with mild impairment has only moderate memory loss, which tends to be more marked for recent events. Professional caregivers should take advantage of the person's ability to express and/or exhibit likes and dislikes and to maintain talents and hobbies, family relationships, and interests. This information can serve as a basis for current and future activity and care plans. Because the person is still aware of his or her needs (even though assistance may be needed to attend to many of them), it is essential to the person's dignity that he or she be included in developing the care plan.

During Stage 1, the person with cognitive impairment may be experiencing extreme frustration as he or she realizes that it is becoming more difficult to accomplish tasks that once were basic. The person is aware of the need for assistance and possibly is discouraged and frightened by the understanding of the drastic changes in the future. These feelings should be addressed, using the utmost care and respect. The resident needs to feel safe and must know that he or she will be treated with dignity throughout the course of the disease. Positive interactions provide the reassurance needed at this time.

The activity program should concentrate on the person's abilities and interests, and the required assistance should be provided to allow the person to experience the greatest amount of success in as many areas as possible. At this stage, individuals usually focus on those tasks that they can no longer accomplish. They are aware of and are sensitive to cognitive losses more at this time than at any other. The professional caregiver should make a tremendous effort to refocus the person's attention toward abilities and strengths.

Even though the activities described in this chapter are within an individual's range of abilities in Stage 1, they may not suit the person's preferences. The person is still able to perform most of the tasks and activities associated with previous routines. Planned activities should blend into a familiar, daily schedule. The resident may feel insulted by being encouraged to participate in activities that were not part of the day before the onset of the disease or that may seem "childish."

An activity hour is usually not appropriate for individuals in the early part of Stage 1. For a person in this stage, activities can mean everyday tasks that are supported through sensitivity to communication deficits and through simplification of complex routines. The flow of the daily routine should remain the same for as long as possible.

The person in Stage 1 may be successful with many activities from before the onset of dementia if consideration is given to the loss of communication skills. Very often, the person understands many spoken or written words and can communicate many thoughts, needs, opinions, and feelings with only slight difficulty. It is common for the individual to "cover up" for what cannot be understood or expressed. The person will often look for and use body language, tone of voice, and demonstration to fill in the gaps.

As many familiar daily activities, routines, and hobbies as are reasonable for people in Stage 1 should be included. An activity should be introduced by breaking it down into manageable steps so as not to overwhelm the individual. When explaining a procedure, the caregiver should use simple, short statements and explanations. Words can be clarified with voice tone, body language, and visual demonstrations. In this way, the person can remain involved in previously familiar activities and routines. This sense of involvement is essential to the person's sense of individuality at this time. Alternative approaches should be considered only when these activities require abilities beyond the person's capacities and/or when they are too frustrating.

Sensory Activities

A person in the first stage of dementia has only moderate difficulty in handling problems or in recognizing similarities and differences. Take advantage of the person's intact strengths by providing a wide variety of sensory activities.

Visual activities focus on discriminating sizes, shapes, colors, numbers, and topical pictures, which builds on existing abilities to recognize similarities and differences. Puzzles and hand–eye integration focus on the existing strengths of problem solving. Recognition and/or comparison of items utilizing the senses of smell, touch, hearing, and taste are also suitable because they employ the same strengths as the visual activities and provide an opportunity to increase the variety of experiences.

Activities of Daily Living

A person in the first stage of dementia exhibits mild but definite impairment of the ability to perform ADLs and often will abandon more difficult chores. Personal care frequently needs prompting, although numerous tasks and activities are still within the person's capabilities. The individual must be allowed and encouraged to participate in as many activities as possible in this category.

Past household responsibilities and/or professions are an excellent guide to determining the most logically suitable activities, although the activities may need to be simplified. Providing for continued experiences in those areas of interest can instill the positive feelings that were previously connected to the performance of such tasks. However, new activities can also be introduced at this stage.

Although prompting may be needed for the older adult to carry out personal care tasks, he or she should be encouraged to perform these basic tasks for as long as possible. The ability to care for one's personal hygiene is basic to one's sense of dignity. To succeed, the person often needs only verbal encouragement and/or the simplification of these tasks. For example, instead of merely telling residents that they need to brush their teeth, they can be gently reminded that they may want to brush their teeth and then show them where the toothbrush and toothpaste are kept. Residents may need step-by-step reminders of the process involved in this task. Residents should be allowed to indicate how much assistance is necessary. The amount of assistance and/or simplification of tasks varies among the different aspects of personal care.

Physical Activities

Physical activities are an excellent diversion in Stage 1, when more time is available as a result of decreasing ability to perform previous activities. Residents still maintain social capabilities at this stage. They will enjoy many of their previous social activities and should be encouraged to do so. Physical activities can relieve frustrations and tensions. Again, use references to the past and familiar routines as a guide in selecting physical tasks, games, and sports. Very often, simply taking a walk fulfills the need to expend energy and provides an opportunity for companionship and conversation.

A person with mild cognitive impairment typically abandons more complicated hobbies. A hobby is often representative of an individual's talents, dreams, or most desired form of relaxation and enjoyment. Most hobbies and special interests can be simplified, so the person should be encouraged and given the opportunity to continue to participate. The person should be presented with less complex tasks to perform rather than with all the steps involved in the project. It is not uncommon, however, for an individual to become angry when given a simplified version of his hobby, especially if that hobby required years of practice to master. The inability to perform at the highest level reveals his or her own deterioration. If this is the case, introducing alternative activities can result in less upset.

ACTIVITIES FOR STAGE 2 OF DEMENTIA

At Stage 2 of dementia, an individual will most likely be seen in a home health program, adult day services, or long-term care setting. Family caregivers who feel overwhelmed by the responsibilities of caring for their loved one turn to professionals for assistance and guidance to cope with the person's increasing needs. An important responsibility for the professional is to train family members and friends in the approach and objectives of positive interactions in order to be able to participate in the individual's care in a more positive way. This training serves not only the person but also the family and staff.

Sensory Activities

Most of the sensory activities are appropriate for the person with moderate cognitive impairment, although they will often need to be simplified. Sensory activities should be introduced at a slower pace, and the caregiver needs to provide a higher degree of encouragement, such as step-by-step demonstration or hand-in-hand assistance.

Visual activities are most likely the best suited for a person in Stage 2. Even though the person is experiencing severe memory loss, he or she retains highly learned material (a memory that has been reinforced constantly). The visual activities call upon existing abilities by using numbers, colors, shapes, and easily identifiable pictures.

Activities that focus on smell, hearing, and taste may require individual modification, because these senses often deteriorate with the normal aging process. Each individual's strengths and preferences relating to these senses should always be taken into account.

Tactile activities using textures, lotions/massage, and animals are usually very comforting and relaxing. Manipulating locks, zippers, buttons, or Velcro tend to be successful activities because most persons in this stage need to keep their hands "busy."

Activities of Daily Living

The person in Stage 2 has the ability to perform only very simple chores. All ADLs are appropriate, as they have already been simplified or can be adjusted in degree of difficulty. For some people, abilities in this area are highly learned, so ADLs are relevant.

The person at this stage often requires a great deal of assistance with personal hygiene and dressing. If these activities are approached as opportunities for positive interaction, the person can still achieve success. A task may be broken down into manageable parts. The caregiver should demonstrate, encourage, and reward at each step. Caring for one's own grooming needs instills a sense of independence and dignity, and every effort should be made to provide opportunities that will help lead a person to this outcome.

Physical Activities

In Stage 2 the person with dementia is disoriented in time and place, often wandering or pacing. When structured throughout the day, physical activities can be a positive means of utilizing this energy. The activities need not be strenuous. Target games, par courses (a walking exercise course with stations along the course at which different exercises and stretches are done), and movement/exercise to music can be successful.

Physical activities work well either as individual or group activities. Groups also provide an opportunity for socialization.

ACTIVITIES FOR STAGE 3 OF DEMENTIA

The person in Stage 3 is most likely cared for in a long-term care facility. Many of the suggested activities in this program would only frustrate him or her, calling upon abilities that have been lost. However, the positive interactions approach remains applicable. Interactions with a person with severe impairment should focus on nurturing and comforting.

Sensory Activities

Because of the person's severe impairment in the area of problem solving, most of the sensory activities involving these abilities (e.g., matching colors, shapes, numbers, textures, flavors) should not be introduced. Looking at pictures or family albums presents an excellent opportunity for the caregiver to spend time with the resident. Listening to music can be very relaxing.

Activities of Daily Living

At this stage, the person is most likely able to attend to very few, if any, personal care needs. He or she is likely to be incontinent. The professional caregiver can attend to these personal care needs while supporting the person's sense of dignity. Brushing the person's hair or gently massaging his or her hands and back with lotion while speaking in a soft tone can be very comforting to the resident. A slow, gentle, nurturing approach can be applied to all aspects of care. Although the person will not understand all words spoken, he or she will understand gentleness and caring expressed through tone and touch.

Physical Activities

The movement of muscles and joints is important at any stage of dementia. However, because an individual in Stage 3 is usually very ill and frail, the amount and type of physical activity are best determined by a physician, nurse, or physical therapist.

GUIDELINES FOR COMMUNICATION

The brain is a magnificent creation. Cognitively healthy individuals can process visual, auditory, tactile, olfactory, and gustatory cues; can process verbal information; and can react and respond. When cognition begins to deteriorate, these processes are delayed, and the person's ability to focus and absorb information becomes inconsistent. Communication must reflect respect for the struggle and should be restructured around this disability.

For many people with cognitive impairment, their word-finding ability has deteriorated to such an extent that even when they seem to know the answer, they cannot "find" the word. Because this is extremely frustrating, as the disease progresses, caregivers need to become increasingly sensitive to the time when questions must be limited.

The Positive Interactions Program slows down and emphasizes every step in processing information to provide the person with the greatest possibility of understanding. Each step is necessary for realizing the objectives of positive interactions.

Nonverbal communication such as body language, voice tone, and facial expression can convey a great amount of information to the older adult with cognitive impairment. As the ability to process verbal information deteriorates, the person becomes increasingly sensitive to nonverbal signals.

Clear communication, verbal and nonverbal alike, is the essence of any successful interaction. The following suggestions will enhance effectiveness in communicating with a person with cognitive impairment.

1. Do not begin talking to the person until he or she is facing you. Say the person's name while touching his or her arm.
2. Speak clearly and in short sentences.
3. Use gestures when appropriate. Point to objects or demonstrate an action, such as brushing your teeth.
4. Provide these individuals with every opportunity to express themselves. If they are concentrating on something, do not speak too soon or they will lose their train of thought. Do not interrupt, even if it takes longer for them to say what they want. They may view your finishing their sentences as a negative statement about their ability to communicate, which may be discouraging.
5. Be a creative listener. Listen for the true meaning. Often you can "hear" the meaning by thinking in metaphor (e.g., mother = care = home = safe).
6. Do not argue over the correct answer. The person may often confuse his or her relatives and may call you "mother" but mean "nurse." Also, remember that the person may be describing his or her reality. If he or she says it is winter even though it is the middle of July, it may feel like, look like, and be what "winter" is for him or her.
7. Use "I" statements as opposed to "you" statements if you do become angry. For example, say "I'm feeling angry. I need to rest now," instead of "You make me so angry that I can't stand to be here." The resident did not cause your bad feelings and cannot change his or her behavior for you. Also, it may be frightening to see you angry when the person feels so helpless. Talk to a colleague when you need to blow off steam.
8. When residents are no longer able to communicate verbally, keep talking to them about those things that were important to them, such

as family members, career, and hobbies. Speak clearly; say the names of people the person loves; touch the person; and massage the person's arms, feet, head, and back. Touch is the greatest communicator.

Check the facilitator's tone of voice, body language, and other outward signs that can be perceived. The person will certainly notice if the facilitator is feeling tired, aggravated, or frustrated, and attempts to communicate will be unsuccessful. The person needs to feel comfortable at his or her level for the program to work effectively. This joint effort will create a new, meaningful way to spend time together. These steps should become a style that is used in all interactions, including routine tasks.

VARIATIONS ON A THEME

The professional training of the activities coordinator will influence the flavor of the Positive Interactions Program. At the Jewish Community Centers Association Adult Day Care Program in St. Louis, Missouri, where this approach was developed, the different staff coordinators over the past 7 years have shown how this interactive plan can be adapted to a variety of professional disciplines.

The Positive Interactions Program was initially implemented through the creativity and passion for excellence exhibited by the entire adult day services staff. The program occupational therapist promoted a design incorporating sensory activities, which held promise for adults with cognitive impairment who had lost their abilities in language, yet were still capable in visual, tactile, and auditory areas. Another staff member focused on the ADLs that could be practiced in the adult day services setting in order to reestablish self-esteem. A coordinator whose graduate degree was in art therapy adapted some of her art projects within the framework of the program, offering a creative and colorful means of self-expression and providing enormous satisfaction and pride to the participants. When the program is designed with the group's skill level in mind, pleasure can be derived from the work as well as the results (e.g., making string art, flower pressing, marble painting, starch painting, decorating and coloring bookmarks and note cards, making collages, material dyeing and printing, embossing paper).

Nurturing, validation, and touch were emphasized when the staff coordinator had training in gerontology and social work. There was a warm, soft environment that exuded calmness. Members of the group gave hand massages to one another, listened to music that used sounds from nature, and experienced group cohesiveness. Varying degrees of attention were given to the "what," but the "how" was always central. The quality of the interaction was the critical focus of each activity variation.

As the program continues under the direction of a recreational therapist, a balance is again struck within the framework of the program. Although success, partnerships, and expressions of respect are the foundation, additional sources of activity development are holistic health, relaxation, and massage techniques; self-affirmation; and validation.

These examples have demonstrated the wide range of emphases that can be woven into a program whose design promotes self-esteem, involvement, and participation in life.

CONCLUSIONS

The goal of successful intervention is to open doors for people who would otherwise be locked out. Addressing individual strengths and designing programs with these strengths in mind is critical to making an impact on individuals with dementia.

Adult day services may have an advantage in that they emphasize activities. The knowledge gained by professionals interacting on a social and recreational level with adults with cognitive impairment has been valuable to the practice of gerontology. Even when there are medical treatments that provide individuals with a sense of hope, helping these adults and their families to cope on a day-to-day basis is crucial. The frustrating lack of medical interventions for people with Alzheimer's disease means that the focus on the quality of life within the psychosocial realm is ever more important.

REFERENCES

Miller, B.A. (1988). Reliability of the Washington University Clinical Dementia Rating, *Archives of Neurology, 45.*

Morris, J. (1993, November). *Neurology, 43*(11), 2413.

Nissenboim, S., & Vroman, C. (1995). *Interactions by design.* St. Louis: Geri-Active Consultants.

APPENDIX

Dusting Furniture/Vacuuming/Sweeping/Washing Windows

Materials

Dust cloth and furniture polish for furniture, vacuum for carpets, broom for sweeping, window cleaner and cloth for windows

These household chores can be approached as activities. They can relieve some of the caregiver's burden while instilling a feeling of usefulness in the person, and they can be incorporated into your daily routine. This will call for a slightly different approach compared with most of the other sensory integration activities because it will be difficult to remove many of the distractions. To limit distraction as much as possible, set up the person with one item at a time to be dusted or one small area to be vacuumed or swept. Because there are several processes to each task, let the person do just one of these processes. It may be difficult for the person to remember sequenced tasks (e.g., it might be preferable for you to spray the furniture polish and he or she wipes it off). It may also be safer if you handle the spray can.

For ease of explanation, the examples used pertain to dusting furniture.

Objectives

1. Provide an opportunity for success.
2. Provide an opportunity for quality time together.
3. Accept the person at his or her level.

Activity and Approaches

1. Familiarize the person with the dust cloth and furniture polish:

   "Here is a can of furniture polish and dust cloth."

2. Describe what you are going to do:

   "Let's dust the furniture together."

3. Demonstrate by dusting a portion of a table, explaining each step:

   "First, I'll spray some of this polish on the table and then I'll wipe it off with this cloth."

4. Encourage and reward the person's participation. It may work out best if you spray the polish and have the person wipe it off:

   "Would you like to help me?"
   "I'll spray and you wipe."
   "You're really doing a nice job, and I appreciate your help."

Appendix adapted from Nissenboim, S., & Vroman, C. (1995). *Interactions by design*. St. Louis: Geri-Active Consultants.

Looking at Topical Pictures

Materials

Groups of pictures related to specific topics (e.g., weddings, babies, animals, weather, sports). Each group should have four to six pictures in it, and the topic should be chosen according to the person's interests and abilities.

The best resources for clear pictures are at a teacher's supply store. Magazine pictures are often too busy. Find pictures that are very basic.

Objectives

1. Provide an opportunity for success.
2. Provide an opportunity for quality time together.
3. Accept the person at his or her level.

Activity and Approaches

1. Familiarize the person with the pictures. Introduce only one topic at a time:

   "Here are some pictures."
2. Name and describe the related pictures:

   "Here is a picture of a bride and groom."
   "Here is a picture of a church."
3. Demonstrate by discussing how the pictures relate to each other. Stimulate specific memories relating to the topic:

   "All these pictures remind me of a wedding."
   "Do you remember your wedding?"
4. Encourage free association. Accept all memories even if they are not associated with the topic. The topic may have triggered another memory—go with the person's associations:

   "Yes, you're right. The bride does look like Alana."

Massaging

Materials

Skin lotion

Objectives

1. Provide an opportunity for success.
2. Provide an opportunity for quality time together.
3. Accept the person at his or her level.

Activity and Approaches

1. Familiarize the person with the lotion by letting him or her handle the container and feel a small amount of the lotion:

   "Here is a container of skin lotion."

2. Explain how and why the lotion is used:

   "This lotion is used to rub into your skin."
   "It makes your skin feel soft and helps heal chapped skin."

3. Demonstrate by placing a small amount of lotion in your hand and massage both of your hands:

   "I'm going to put a little of the lotion in the palm of my hand and then rub it in like this."

4. Encourage the person to do the same. Take turns massaging each other's hands. Touching hands in a gentle manner can be very relaxing and rewarding:

   "Let me put a little lotion in the palm of your hand and you rub it in like I just did."
   "Doesn't the lotion make your hands feel good?"

Matching Textures Through Touch

Materials

Four or five pairs of material swatches. The swatches should be of distinctly different textures (e.g., two swatches of silk, two swatches of burlap, two swatches of wool, two swatches of suede).

Objectives

1. Provide an opportunity for success.
2. Provide an opportunity for quality time together.
3. Accept the person at his or her level.

Activity and Approaches

1. Familiarize the person with the swatches of material by letting him or her handle each one:

   "Here are some pieces of material."

2. Name the materials and describe the textures of each. Also, emphasize that there are two swatches of each texture:

   "Here are two pieces of silk."
   "Feel how soft they are."

3. Demonstrate by selecting one of the swatches and, after touching each of the other pieces of material, selecting the appropriate match. Explain why the other materials are not the correct match as you feel them:

   "Here's a piece of burlap."
   "It feels rough."
   "I am going to feel all the other pieces of material and see if I can find one that feels just like this burlap."
   "This piece doesn't feel like the burlap because it feels soft."

4. Encourage and reward participation. Discuss the clothing the person wears that is made of the same fabrics:

"Here is a piece of wool."
"Feel it and then see if you can find another piece of material that feels the same."
"Yes, you're right. It does feel scratchy."
"Sweaters are sometimes made of wool."

Playing Ball Games/Balloon Games

Materials

One medium to large soft rubber ball, a balloon, or a beach ball

This activity is particularly enjoyable for most people. It should be fun, simple, a great outlet for energy, and a good form of exercise. There are many variations of these activities. They can be done sitting or standing, but they should be set up in an area with sufficient space to prevent breaking anything. Some of the activities that have been found to be successful are bouncing the ball back and forth, hitting the balloon to each other, and kicking the ball to each other. These activities can provide a good opportunity for positive interaction between the person and a younger child, such as a grandchild. It is also a great group activity. When you are going to involve another person in an activity, you may need to start the activity by following the usual steps of familiarizing, describing, demonstrating, and encouraging before removing yourself from the activity. You may also need to encourage the third person, especially a child, because he or she may be uncomfortable at first with the interaction. For the ease of explanation, the examples used pertain to bouncing the ball back and forth between the person and a grandchild.

Objectives

1. Provide an opportunity for success.
2. Provide an opportunity for quality time together.
3. Accept the person at his or her level.

Activity and Approaches

1. Familiarize the person with the ball by letting him or her handle it:

   "Here is a red rubber ball."

2. Describe what you are going to do:

   "Michael would like to play ball with you."
   "There is plenty of room if you sit here and Michael stands over here."
   "We're going to bounce the ball to each other."

3. Demonstrate by bouncing the ball back and forth as you explain what you are doing:

   "Okay, Michael, I'm going to bounce the ball to you."
   "Good catch."

"Now you bounce it back to me."
"Great!"

4. Encourage and reward participation:

   "Now it's Grandpa's turn."
   "You bounce it to Michael."
   "That's great!"
   "You two look like you're having fun together."

Playing Target Games

Materials

Four or five small soft balls or four or five beanbags and a small trash can or basket. Other target games that can be utilized are Velcro dart boards, foam rubber basketballs, bowling and similar games currently available at toy/game stores.

Most people find this activity particularly enjoyable. It should be fun, simple, a great outlet for energy, and a good form of exercise. This activity can also provide a good opportunity for positive interaction between the person and a younger child, such as a grandchild. When you are going to involve another person in an activity, you may need to start the activity by following the usual steps of familiarizing, describing, demonstrating, and encouraging before you remove yourself from the activity. You may also need to encourage the third person, especially a child, because he or she may be uncomfortable at first with the interaction.

Objectives

1. Provide an opportunity for success.
2. Provide an opportunity for quality time together.
3. Accept the person at his or her level.

Activity and Approaches

1. Familiarize the person with the beanbags and the basket by letting him or her handle the beanbags:

   "Here are four beanbags and a basket."

2. Describe what you are going to do:

   "Jennifer would like to play a game with you."
   "We'll take turns throwing the beanbags into the basket."

3. Demonstrate by throwing the beanbags into the basket as you explain what you are doing:

   "Jennifer, you go first."
   "Throw one of your beanbags into the basket."
   "You made it! That's great!"

4. Encourage and reward participation:

   "Now it's Grandpa's turn."

"Here's a beanbag for you."
"Try and throw it into the basket."
"You made it too."
"You guys are too good for me."

Setting the Table

Materials

Place mats, unbreakable plates, silverware, and napkins

Before beginning this activity, break it down into manageable parts. For example, first familiarize, name, and demonstrate only the place mats. When the person has completed that step, then familiarize, name, and demonstrate the plates and other objects. Be sure to reward the person for all attempts.

Because it will take much more time to allow the person to help you set the table and you will have to be there for each step, be sure to begin well in advance of actually needing the table to be set.

Objectives

1. Provide an opportunity for success.
2. Provide an opportunity for quality time together.
3. Accept the person at his or her level.

Activity and Approaches

1. Familiarize the person with the items he or she will be working with:

   "Here are four place mats."

2. Briefly explain what you will be doing:

   "Vern and Bernard are coming for dinner tonight, so we need to set the table."
   "I'd like you to set the table with me."

3. Demonstrate by showing the person what you want him or her to do:

   "Let's put a place mat in front of each chair."
   "I'll put this one here."

4. Encourage and reward participation:

   "Now you put this place mat right over there."
   "Very good."
   "I really appreciate your help."
   "The boys will also be happy that you did such a nice job."
   "Now let's put the plates on the table."

Sorting Laundry

Materials

Two or three laundry baskets, laundry that needs to be washed, or laundry that has already been washed and dried.

To eliminate distraction, have the person sort the laundry into general categories first (e.g., socks, towels, shirts). Then from the general categories, sort into specific categories (e.g., bath towels, hand towels). Present the person with only one general category at a time.

Objectives

1. Provide an opportunity for success.
2. Provide an opportunity for quality time together.
3. Accept the person at his or her level.

Activity and Approaches

1. Familiarize the person with the laundry baskets and the laundry:
   "Here are some baskets and some clean laundry."
2. Name the different items of laundry:
   "Here is a towel."
   "Here is a sock."
3. Demonstrate by sorting the laundry into categories. Explain what you are doing as you are sorting:
   "Let's sort the laundry together."
   "We'll put all the towels in this basket and all the socks in this basket."
   "Here's a towel, so I'll put it in here."
4. Encourage and reward participation:
   "Here's another towel."
   "You put it in the basket with the other towels."
   "You're doing a great job, and I appreciate your help."

Walking

Materials

No materials necessary

Taking walks is a great way to release energy. It also provides an opportunity for quiet time together. There may be certain times during the day when the person regularly becomes agitated. If so, you can schedule a walk before this time in hopes of decreasing or eliminating this agitated behavior. The person may also need to walk after sitting for a period of time with other activities of this program. For some, walking may be viewed as a reward for completing these activities. The time and duration of the walk will depend on your schedule and on the person's behavior and endurance.

Objectives

1. Provide an opportunity for success.
2. Provide an opportunity for quality time together.
3. Accept the person at his or her level.

Activity and Approaches

Because this is not an activity like others in the program, there are no formal steps to follow. You should still familiarize and describe to the person what you are going to do and where you will be walking. Encouragement and reward are always necessary. The main purpose of the walk is exercise, but you should also enjoy the time together. Something the person sees or hears during the walk may stimulate a pleasant memory for him or her.

4

Clinical Issues in Advanced Dementia

Ladislav Volicer, M.D., Ph.D.

Alzheimer's disease is the most common cause of progressive dementia in older adults (Breteler, Claus, Van Duijn, Launer, & Hofman, 1992). The prevalence of Alzheimer's disease increases with age, from 10% in individuals over the age of 65 to 47% in individuals over the age of 85 (Evans et al., 1989). Life expectancy in the United States has increased, and people over 85 years old represent the fastest-growing segment of the population. Alzheimer's disease thus affects increasing numbers of people and is taking on increasing importance.

Definitive diagnosis of Alzheimer's disease requires examination of the brain tissue obtained during autopsy. Its clinical picture is often difficult to distinguish from other progressive dementias, such as Pick's disease, multi-infarct dementia, and diffuse Lewy body disease. Moreover, often autopsy finds a combination of two or more of these conditions, especially of multi-infarct and Lewy bodies with Alzheimer plaques and tangles. Because the dementing process is irreversible in all these conditions, the clinical management is similar in middle- and late-stage dementia regardless of its etiology. Therefore, although this chapter mainly deals with

Alzheimer's disease, the same considerations apply to other progressive dementias.

COURSE OF ALZHEIMER'S DISEASE

Alzheimer's disease develops insidiously and can be seen as a gradual loss of independence (Figure 4.1). The first symptoms of the disease are usually memory problems or disorientation in familiar surroundings. However, some people develop mood or personality changes before their memory problems are recognized. In the early stage people with dementia are still able to care for themselves and to engage in leisure activities. In the middle stage people with dementia require constant supervision, lose the ability to use common household utensils, and develop speech difficulties and incontinence. Late-stage Alzheimer's disease is characterized by motor difficulties leading to inability to walk, chew, and sometimes swallow. Individuals become completely dependent on their caregivers in all activities of daily living (ADLs). From first symptoms to death the average duration of Alzheimer's disease is 8 years, with large variability in the rate of disease progression (Volicer et al., 1987).

BEHAVIORAL PROBLEMS

Four main behavioral syndromes occur in the middle and late stages of dementia: depression, sleep disturbances, agitation, and resistiveness.

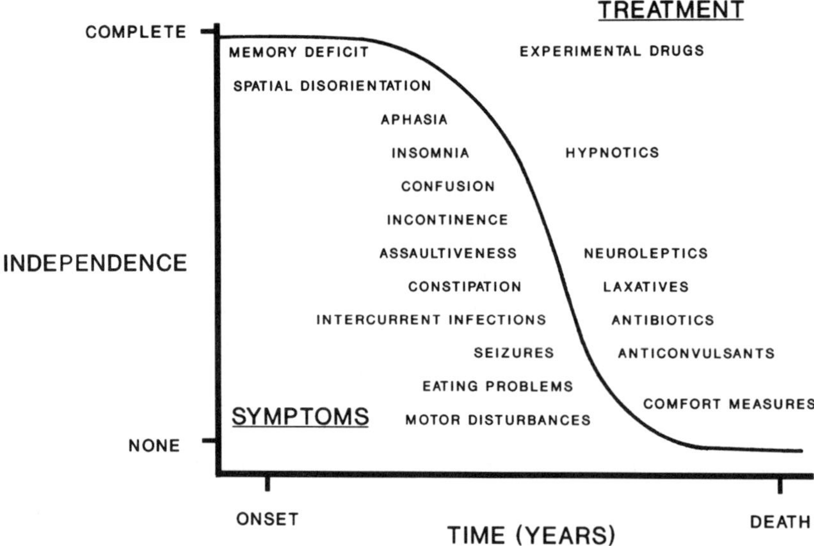

Figure 4.1. Course of Alzheimer's disease.

Depression

The diagnosis of depression in people with dementia is difficult because six of eight symptoms of major depressive disorder (four of which are required for diagnosis according to the *Diagnostic and Statistical Manual of Mental Disorders*, 4th ed. [DSM-IV; American Psychiatric Association, 1994]) are commonly seen in the middle and late stages of dementia (i.e., poor appetite or weight loss; sleep disturbance; fatigue; psychomotor agitation or retardation; loss of interest in usual activities; diminished ability to think and concentrate). Depressed mood, the major criterion of depression, appears less frequently but may be difficult to assess because of the individual's aphasia and cognitive impairment (Lazarus, Newton, Cohler, Lesser, & Schwein, 1987). It is not surprising, therefore, that estimates of coexistent depression in dementia vary widely, ranging from 0% to 86% (Wragg & Jeste, 1989). Dementia and depression may represent two extremes of a continuum, with frequent combination of both disorders (Emery & Oxman, 1992).

Treatment of depression in people with dementia is important because it improves mood, vegetative signs, and ADLs in as many as 85% of people with dementia (Reifler, Larson, Teri, & Poulsen, 1986). The diagnosis must rely on nonverbal cues, such as sad facial expression, food refusal, and crying spells. Sometimes angry expression and hostile behavior are signs of depression, which improves after antidepressant treatment. Although tricyclic antidepressants are effective, their use in people with dementia is limited by their anticholinergic (e.g., dryness of mouth, difficulty urinating) and cardiovascular (e.g., decreased blood pressure, cardiac arrhythmia) side effects. Drugs that act more specifically on the serotoninergic system (e.g., trazodone, sertraline) are well tolerated and are effective in improving mood in people with late-stage dementia.

Disturbances of the Sleep–Wake Cycle

Alzheimer's disease leads to cell loss in the suprachiasmatic nucleus of the hypothalamus, which regulates circadian rhythms (rhythmic repetition of certain phenomena in living organisms at about the same time every 24 hours) (Swaab, Fliers, & Partiman, 1985). This cell loss may be the cause of sleep–wake cycle disturbances, which almost all individuals develop in middle- and/or late-stage dementia. These people have more awakenings from sleep and less slow-wave and REM sleep than do controls (Bliwise, 1993; Vitiello & Prinz, 1989). A correlation exists between sleep disruption and severity of dementia in people with middle- and late-stage dementia (Vitiello, Bliwise, & Prinz, 1992). Many people with dementia also develop a routine of frequent daytime naps with prolonged periods of nighttime wakefulness (Vitiello et al., 1992). In a person still living at home and cared for by family members, this sleep reversal makes provision of care difficult because it deprives the caregiver of sleep.

Treatment of sleep–wake cycle disturbances is difficult. Nonpharmacological treatment is preferable but is not always effective. This treatment includes avoidance of daytime napping by keeping people occupied by activities, establishing a regular nighttime routine, and possibly providing nighttime activities for people who are awake (Bliwise, 1993). Interventions that improve circadian rhythm may be also useful because exposure to bright light has been shown to improve sleep in individuals with dementia (Satlin, Volicer, Ross, Herz, & Campbell, 1992).

Benzodiazepine hypnotics (e.g., temazepam) are effective in inducing sleep, but they must be given for a prolonged period of time in people with dementia, often resulting in the development of tolerance to the drug. Chloralhydrate is an older hypnotic that is effective and affects the sleep stages less. However, it may be related to agitation in the afternoon and evening of the following day (sundowning) (Little, Satlin, Sunderland, & Volicer, 1995). Diphenhydramine is a sedating antihistamine that is useful as a hypnotic. It has anticholinergic activity (Hirschowitz & Molina, 1988), which may aggravate memory problems, but this effect may be less important in late-stage dementia, when cognitive losses are severe. A newer hypnotic, zolpidem, which acts on benzodiazepine receptors but affects the sleep stages less, may be useful in treating insomnia. Sedating antidepressants (e.g., trazodone, doxepin) are good alternative agents, especially for a person with some depressive symptomatology.

Agitation

Restlessness and pacing occur often in middle- and late-stage dementia. Agitation makes provision of care for individuals with dementia more difficult because it increases resistiveness to care (see next section). Restless patients may not be willing to participate in any activities or even to sit down for meals. The cause of agitation is difficult to identify and may vary in different people. In some people with dementia it may be an expression of anxiety, provoked, for instance, by a visit from family members or by hallucinations and delusions. In some individuals agitation may be an expression of fatigue; some evidence indicates that people with dementia are less tolerant of the stress of daily activities (Hall, 1993). Agitation may also be related to disturbances of the circadian rhythms described earlier. Sundowning appears in some people (Bliwise, 1993), and others are more agitated in the morning (Cohen-Mansfield, Werner, & Marx, 1989).

The best management strategies for agitation are environmental modifications. Avoiding the simultaneous visit of numerous relatives, noise, and activities that the individual cannot comprehend help prevent agitated behavior. A safe environment in which the person can walk unsupervised provides opportunity for exercise, which also helps decrease agitation. Drug treatment may be necessary if agitation interferes with eating or provision of care or if it is an expression of the person's discomfort. Short-acting benzodiazepines (e.g., lorazepam) are effective in decreasing agitation when anxiety is the provoking stimulus. However, some individuals develop a paradoxical stimulation and increased confusion shortly after benzodiazepine administration, and tolerance to benzodiazepines may develop. Diphenhydramine provides mild daytime sedation without paradoxical stimulation and tolerance/dependence, and its anticholinergic effect may not be significant in individuals whose memory is already severely impaired. Buspirone may be also helpful, but must be given in sufficiently large doses (up to 60 mg/day), and the onset of its effect is delayed. Neuroleptic therapy is indicated if agitation is caused by hallucinations or delusions (see later in this chapter).

Resistiveness

Although some people with Alzheimer's disease sometimes strike out, this rarely happens without some external stimulus. Most of these individuals are content when left alone and may not comprehend that an ADL is necessary. Because of their confusion, they do not cooperate with care and may actually resist it. If the caregiver insists, the resistiveness may escalate into combative behavior, resulting in an assault (Figure 4.2). Because of this escalation sequence, the best treatment consists of prevention of resistive behavior by adapting nursing strategies. For instance, it may be effective not to insist on performing an activity but to leave and come back a few minutes later, after the person has forgotten the episode and may be more amenable to care. Another strategy is employing two caregivers, one who distracts the person and the other who provides the care.

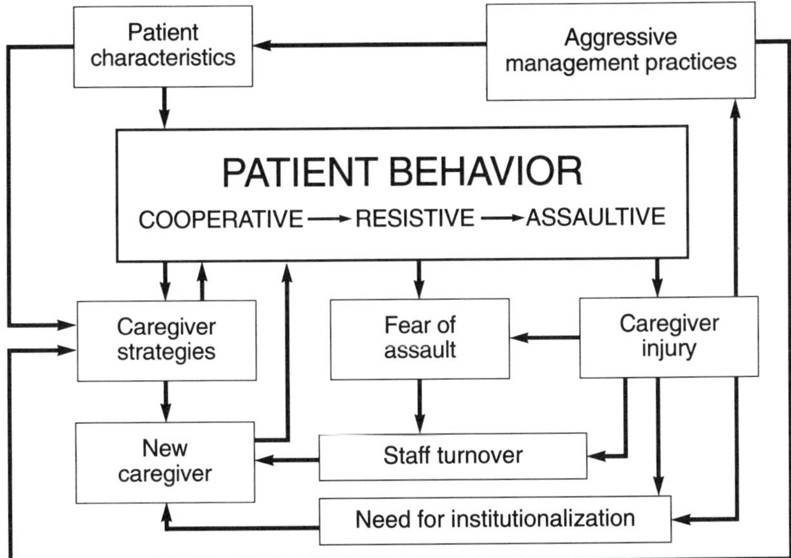

Figure 4.2. Resistive behavior of individuals with Alzheimer's disease.

For many individuals, however, these strategies may not be sufficient. The person's resistiveness may be accentuated by hallucinations or delusions, often with paranoid content. In these cases treatment with neuroleptics may be necessary. Although information from well-controlled drug studies is limited, all neuroleptics seem to be equally effective in decreasing resistive behavior and are more effective than benzodiazepines and diphenhydramine (Herz, Volicer, Ross, & Rheaume, 1992). The choice of neuroleptic should be based on the side effect profile; the drug chosen should be the one least likely to produce side effects in the particular individuals. Neuroleptics can be classified on a continuum, with one extreme consisting of drugs possessing the potential for extrapyramidal side effects but not sedative or cardiovascular side effects (e.g., haloperidol, fluphenazine) and the other extreme consisting of drugs having more sedative effect and potential for hypotension and arrhythmias but less potential for extrapyramidal side effects (e.g., thioridazine, molindone). Some drugs have a mixed side effect profile (e.g., thiothixene, perphenazine). A newer neuroleptic, risperidone, has fewer extrapyramidal and cardiovascular side effects than other neuroleptics but has a long half-life that requires very gradual dose adjustment.

The Omnibus Budget Reconciliation Act (OBRA) of 1987 mandates that the drug regimens of all residents in long-term care facilities be free of unnecessary pharmacotherapeutic agents. "Unnecessary" refers to excessive doses of medications for excessive periods of time without adequate monitoring or medications administered in the absence of a diagnosis or appropriate reason for the drug. Specific conditions that justify the use of neuroleptic medication include "organic mental syndromes (including dementia) with associated psychotic and/or agitated features," as defined by behaviors that present danger to the resident and others, and/or interfere with the ability of the staff to provide care. Thus, documented resistiveness is clearly an appropriate reason for neuroleptic treatment, although it must be differentiated from "uncooperativeness," which cannot be used as justification for neuroleptic treatment.

ELIMINATION PROBLEMS

Most people develop incontinence in the middle stage of Alzheimer's disease. As the disease progresses and the person's mobility is impaired, most individuals also develop constipation.

Incontinence

As people with dementia lose their ability to orient themselves, they may become unable to find the bathroom. This may lead initially to urination in inappropriate places, which could be managed by taking the person to a toilet at frequent intervals. People with dementia may also become incontinent during the night, when their confusion is increased. Eventually the person is unable to use the toilet even if taken there and becomes doubly incontinent. In an ambulatory person incontinence is best managed by adult incontinence pads during the day and a condom catheter during the night. As people become unable to walk, condom catheters could also be used during the day, if tolerated.

Constipation

Decreased mobility and especially confinement to bed induces constipation in most individuals with Alzheimer's disease. Constipation may be managed initially by dietary modification, for example, increasing the amount of fiber and using prune juice as a mild stimulant. Very often, however, individuals require additional treatment. Stool softeners, such as docusate sodium (Colace), are sometimes used but are not very effective. In addition, liquid docusate sodium, which must be used if the person is unable to swallow a capsule, has an aversive taste. More effective are osmotic laxatives, such as milk of magnesia and lactulose. Lactulose is especially convenient because it is liquid and has a sweet taste, which makes it readily acceptable to most people. If osmotic laxatives do not achieve adequate elimination, stimulant laxatives such as bisacodyl (Dulcolax) or saline enemas (e.g., Fleet) must be used. The goal is to avoid stool impaction, which might require manual disimpaction.

MANAGEMENT OF INTERCURRENT DISEASES

Because most individuals with Alzheimer's disease are older, they are likely to have other diseases in addition to Alzheimer's disease. In addition, the impairments resulting from middle- and late-stage Alzheimer's disease predispose people to additional conditions. These diseases should not be managed without considering the presence of Alzheimer's disease because of the impact of dementia on the person's response to treatment and because of decreased life expectancy.

Modification of Treatment Modalities

Medical treatments for other coexisting diseases should be modified relatively early in the course of Alzheimer's disease. Individuals with Alzheimer's disease lose the ability to report symptoms and therefore are at increased risk for development of adverse treatment responses. For instance, it is counterproductive to strive for low blood glucose levels in a person with Alzheimer's disease who has diabetes because of the increased danger of hypoglycemic reactions. The treatment of hypertension should not be aggressive because of the person's inability to report hypotensive episodes, which could lead to falls and injuries.

Another consideration is the amount of discomfort associated with a treatment. Because people with dementia do not understand the reason for a medical procedure, even a routine intervention such as blood drawing could lead to agitation and a large degree of discomfort. Therefore, it is important to weigh the costs and benefits of any therapeutic procedure for a person with advanced dementia.

Because Alzheimer's disease shortens the life span, some interventions designed to reduce the long-term risk factors of other disorders may be inappropriate. Inappropriate interventions include the treatment of moderately increased cholesterol levels by a restrictive diet or hypocholesterolemic agents and tight control of blood sugar level and blood pressure.

Some interventions are less likely to be successful in a person suffering from Alzheimer's disease than in an individual with intact brain function. The success rate of resuscitation in individuals with brain impairment, for example, is very low (Applebaum, King, & Finucane, 1990). Furthermore, if successful, resuscitation may cause injuries and requires intensive care, including intravenous lines and a respirator, which can cause considerable discomfort in the person. In addition, cardiac or respiratory arrest always leads to faster progression of dementia, resulting in greater impairment of individuals successfully resuscitated (Applebaum et al., 1990). Therefore, cardiopulmonary resuscitation may not be appropriate in a person with middle- or late-stage Alzheimer's disease.

Management of Infections

Alzheimer's disease affects mainly the areas of the brain involved in memory, speech, and other higher brain functions and does not affect the brain areas that regulate basic body functions, such as breathing and circulation. Therefore, people do not die because of Alzheimer's disease itself, but from its complications.

The progression of Alzheimer's disease invariably leads to incontinence, which predisposes individuals to developing urinary tract infections. This tendency is aggravated by enlargement of the prostate gland in men. The incidence of pneumonia is increased by immobility in people who are no longer able to walk and who become bedridden, and by eating difficulties, which sometimes lead to aspiration. Most individuals die of pneumonia, which some call "the old man's best friend."

Effectiveness of Antibiotic Therapy Although infections may be treated with antibiotics even in a long-term care setting, this may not always be appropriate. The determination of which antibiotic should be used requires invasive diagnostic procedures, such as drawing blood and suctioning sputum, which inflict discomfort. Because these individuals are unable to provide information about their symptoms, any elevation in temperature may need to be considered a sign of infection. This can lead to repeated diagnostic procedures, which identify a source of infection in only two thirds of cases (Fabiszewski, Volicer, & Volicer, 1990). In addition, intramuscular antibiotic administration is painful, and any antibiotic could cause an adverse drug reaction, such as severe diarrhea or suppression of white blood cell formation.

In addition to the complications of antibiotic treatment, diagnosing and treating with antibiotics has been shown to be ineffective in extending life in people with late-stage dementia (Fabiszewski, Volicer, & Volicer, 1990). Fabiszewski et al. (1990) have found that individuals with late-stage dementia had the same life expectancy whether they were treated with antibiotics or given only palliative care (Figure 4.3). In such individuals, even when infections are successfully treated, they usually recur after antibiotics are stopped. New infections may be caused by microbes resistant to the original antibiotic, requiring treatment with other potentially more toxic drugs.

Impact of Treatment on Personal Comfort Another consideration in the management of individuals with advanced Alzheimer's disease is increased discomfort induced by even relatively routine therapeutic interventions. Development of an infection, such as pneumonia, may result in the admission of a person with Alzheimer's disease to an acute care setting from home or from a nursing facility. Most individuals respond poorly to such a change because they become confused by the new environment and staff. An acute care hospital is not equipped to care for patients who might wander at night, try to remove their intravenous lines, or become combative during routine caregiving activities they cannot understand. Too often these problems are managed by physical or chemical restraints that inflict a considerable degree of discomfort.

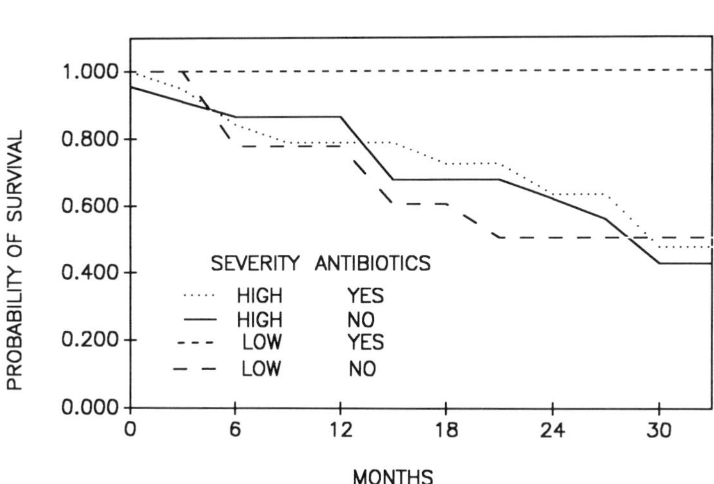

Figure 4.3. Mortality rate of individuals with Alzheimer's disease divided according to language ability and use of antibiotics during a fever episode.

A study conducted on a special care program for people with dementia actually showed that people with dementia exhibited no difference in their observed discomfort before, during, or after an infectious episode regardless of whether they were treated aggressively with antibiotics or were managed palliatively with antipyretics and analgesics (Hurley, Volicer, Mahoney, & Volicer, 1993). Therefore, it may be preferable in the later stages of the dementing disease to avoid admissions to the acute care setting and to provide treatment in long-term care settings. Some aggressive treatment strategies may not be available in long-term care settings but can be replaced by intensive nursing care to ensure comfort—"high touch" instead of "high tech."

MOTOR DIFFICULTIES

In the middle stage of Alzheimer's disease some people become hyperactive and pace most of the time. In the late stage people become unable to walk or to feed themselves and eventually become bedridden. They may also develop contractures and swallowing difficulties.

Ambulation

Pacing significantly increases energy expenditure. Some individuals walk constantly, not even stopping for food, unless they are forced to rest. They may require up to 1,600 Kcal/day more than usual to maintain metabolic balance (Rheaume, Riley, & Volicer, 1987). Constant walking may lead to foot injuries and requires comfortable shoes, preferably walking shoes or sneakers.

As the disease progresses, individuals lose their ability to walk. Some develop gait disturbances, a tendency to lean to one side, leg scissoring, or loss of balance. Others are able to walk, but do not recognize obstacles in their way and walk into walls, furniture, or other people. Because of the potential for injury, these individuals may be able to walk only with assistance. Eventually, they lose their ability to stand and are confined to bed and/or wheelchair.

Muscle Rigidity and Contractures

The combination of Parkinson's disease and Alzheimer's disease is sometimes found during autopsy and may be responsible for the muscle rigidity observed in some individuals with Alzheimer's disease. Alternatively, muscle rigidity could be a side effect of neuroleptic treatment (extrapyramidal [outside the system that controls skilled movements] side effects). Rigidity induced by neuroleptics responds well to anticholinergic therapy, such as benztropine (Cogentin), or to substitution of a neuroleptic with less extrapyramidal side-effect potential, such as thioridazine (Mellaril).

Some individuals in late-stage dementia develop severe muscle contractures (shortening of muscles). Contractures could affect both upper and lower extremities, including fingers, and make provision of nursing care difficult. Finger contractures could lead to palm injury from the fingernails and require protective hand devices. The contractures may be precipitated by immobility in a bedridden or chairbound person. However, contractures do not occur in all individuals and may also be related to extrapyramidal involvement.

EATING DIFFICULTIES

Two main types of eating difficulties can be distinguished: food refusal and swallowing difficulties.

Food Refusal

Refusal of food and liquids is a common problem in management of individuals with advanced dementia of the Alzheimer's type admitted to a hospital or residing in a long-term care facility (Volicer et al., 1989). In most cases the refusal is only occasional and may be managed by changes in diet composition and texture or by the use of dietary supplements (Riley & Volicer, 1990). In some cases refusal of food and liquids results in dehydration and malnutrition and is often managed by the use of enteral tube feeding (Volicer, Rheaume, Riley, Karner, & Glennon, 1990).

The causes of food refusal are difficult to determine. The refusal may involve dislike of institutional food, failure to recognize edible objects as food, or loss of sense of thirst and/or hunger, but it may also be a symptom of depression. Despite diagnostic uncertainty, individuals may benefit from antidepressant treatment (Reifler, Larson, Teri, & Paulsen, 1986).

Swallowing Difficulties

Swallowing difficulties that could lead to aspiration and/or compromised nutritional status pose an additional management dilemma. They may be managed by enteral tube feeding, but tube feeding does not decrease the risk of aspiration in people with swallowing difficulties because it does not prevent the aspiration of respiratory secretions. Adequate nutrition can be maintained by skillful handfeeding and adjustments to diet (Volicer et al., 1989), completely avoiding tube feeding. In addition, tube feeding deprives the person of tasting food and of interacting with the staff during the feeding process, and it increases the person's discomfort and often requires restraints in order to prevent tube removal. Gastrostomy tube feeding may cause less discomfort but requires surgery and may lead to tube migration, the development of granulation tissue and leakage around the stoma, tubal obstruction, diarrhea, nausea, vomiting, abdominal distress, and cramping. Even when adequate calories and protein are provided by the gastrostomy feeding, weight loss may occur (Henderson, Trumbore, Mobarhan, Benya, & Miles, 1992).

Modification of the diet allows oral feeding even in late-stage Alzheimer's disease. A special adult pureed diet has been developed to facilitate the feeding process (Warden, 1989). This diet is low in volume and is nutrient dense. Choking on thin liquids may be managed by using thick liquids, such as yogurt, or by thickening thin liquids with other foods or commercial thickeners (e.g., Thickit). Using these strategies and skillful nursing care, adequate nutrition can be provided even in the terminal stage of Alzheimer's disease. Individuals who are receiving tube feeding should be evaluated and an attempt should be made to convert tube feeding into natural feeding. Such a conversion could significantly improve the person's quality of life and is possible for a large proportion of people with late-stage Alzheimer's disease (Volicer et al., 1990).

TREATMENT STRATEGIES

Because every treatment inflicts a burden on the person being treated, there is a need to compare the benefits and burdens of each treatment to decide which treatment is justified. This comparison is sometimes made paternalistically by the health care provider, who decides for the person what is in his or her best interest. However, it is recognized that the person has a right to accept or refuse a treatment, and respect for the individual's autonomy is generally accepted as an important ethical principle. People suffering from advanced Alzheimer's disease do not, however, have the capacity to understand treatment options and to make informed decisions. Nevertheless, they should not be exposed to a burdensome treatment that may provide little benefit, just because they cannot refuse it. Therefore, a process is needed by which treatment decisions can be made. In some cases this process involves court proceedings, which are cumbersome and time consuming. In most situations, however, a court-appointed guardian or next-of-kin is asked to make treatment decisions. The process of decision making implemented in the author's special care program is summarized in Figure 4.4.

Making such decisions is difficult when individuals have not given clear evidence of their preferences. Most people with dementia do not express clear directives before becoming demented, although in some cases the family could infer the person's wishes from past actions, such as dealing with his or her own aging parents or relatives. In any case, family members must take into consideration the person's conditions, which they are best qualified to compare to the individual's premorbid personality and lifestyle and their own philosophy, which is likely similar to the person's philosophy. However, even taking all these factors into consideration, family members often have difficulty making what could be perceived as life-and-death decisions. This is especially true for some institutionalized individuals whose family members may feel guilty about their inability to care for the person at home. These guilt feelings can be explored and alleviated by discussions in family support groups, and, in addition, caregivers can support family members by holding a conference with the family and recommending an optimal management strategy.

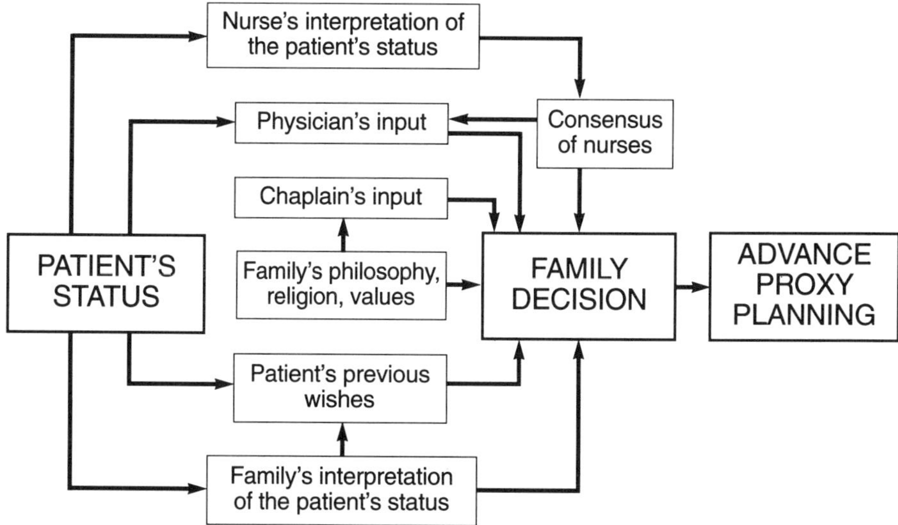

Figure 4.4. Decision-making process for advance proxy planning.

The group that contributes the most important information to the recommendation to the family is the nursing staff, the members of which get to know the person most intimately after admission for long-term care. The consensus of the nursing staff is sought at a meeting of the nursing staff and the attending physician. This meeting occurs shortly before a meeting of the family members with the interdisciplinary team. The meeting with the family members, which is usually chaired by a social worker, provides an opportunity to answer any questions the family might have regarding care and to present staff recommendations about optimal management strategies for the family's consideration. These recommendations are usually presented by the attending physician, who explains the burdens and benefits of each treatment option. Throughout the meeting it is emphasized that the goal of the program is assurance of maximal comfort and that treatment limitation does not mean lack of attention to the person's needs.

A chaplain is also an important member of the interdisciplinary team. The chaplain provides advice regarding the morality of different management options and generally supports the staff recommendations. The chaplain is selected according to the family's religious preferences.

Levels of Care

The staff recommendations deal mainly with clinical decisions that might be necessary at a future date, such as advance proxy planning. Staff members generally find it easier to discuss possible complications before they occur rather than to try to reach a decision in a crisis situation. If the person has a medical problem in addition to Alzheimer's disease, it is also discussed. For example, if a person with Alzheimer's disease has occult gastrointestinal bleeding or he or she may have cancer, the desirability of an extensive diagnostic work-up and treatment would be considered. The advance proxy planning decision consigns the person into one of five levels of care.

The first level represents complete care, including aggressive work-up and treatment of any complication and cardiopulmonary resuscitation (CPR) in case of cardiac or respiratory arrest. The second level eliminates the use of CPR, but maintains all other treatment options. The third level eliminates CPR and transfer to an acute care medical unit for treatment of life-threatening infections, transfusions, or other aggressive interventions. This level eliminates intravenous treatment, use of respirators, and cardiac monitoring. However, a transfer for treatment of an acute complication that is necessary to increase a person's comfort, such as transfer for treatment of a hip fracture, is retained. If clinically indicated, oral or intramuscular antibiotics are used. Hydration is achieved by oral administration of fluids and, if necessary, by short-term nasogastric tube insertion. Avoidance of transfer to an acute care setting aims to prevent exposure of the person to unfamiliar surroundings and caregivers, increased use of restraints, and development of pressure ulcers, which are observed frequently after hospitalization of people in an acute care setting.

The fourth level of care eliminates CPR and transfer to an acute medical unit as well as diagnostic work-up for fevers and treatment of life-threatening infections with antibiotics. However, antibiotics are used if treatment would improve the person's level of comfort, such as in cases of cellulitis (infection of soft tissue by strep and staph bacteria) or cystitis with dysuria (inflammation of the bladder with painful or difficult urination). The fifth level of care eliminates all treatment options listed for the fourth level and, in addition, the use of tubes for artificial nutrition and hydration. Individuals at this level of care are fed orally as much as they can tolerate it, and eating difficulties are minimized by dietary adjustments and intensive nursing care. Analgesics such as acetaminophen or morphine are used liberally for all care levels to ensure comfort.

Hospice Programs

Because there is no known effective treatment that can stop or reverse the progression of Alzheimer's disease, a person in the advanced stage of the disease can be considered terminally ill and similar to a person with incurable cancer. This consideration shifts the emphasis from keeping the person alive at all costs to ensuring comfort. A management strategy concentrating on the individual's comfort is at the heart of the hospice movement, and many people with Alzheimer's disease would benefit from being involved in a hospice program. However, their involvement is complicated by two factors. The first is the inability of people with dementia to make decisions for themselves; the second is the difficulty of predicting the duration of survival.

The process of deciding for or against a hospice program could be the same as that described here for assigning individuals to a level of care. Hospice care is now available for Medicare recipients with terminal diseases when the anticipated survival time is certified by a physician and a hospice director as being 6 months or less, if the disease runs its normal course. However, the variable rate of deterioration in Alzheimer's disease makes it difficult to make an informed judgment about anticipated survival time. Therefore, people with Alzheimer's disease are not generally certified as eligible for coverage for hospice programs under Medicare.

The late stage of Alzheimer's disease may last 1–3 years, and even longer in some people. It is difficult to predict survival on the basis of the severity of dementia alone because death is not directly related to disease progression but to the occurrence of complications. However, it is possible to estimate the probability of death occurring within 6 months if a person's risk factors are considered at the time when a fever indicating the onset of an infection occurs (Volicer, Hurley, Fabiszewski, Montgomery, & Volicer, 1993). Analysis of the mortality pattern of individuals with Alzheimer's disease cared for in two long-term care settings indicated that their survival was statistically associated with age, severity of Alzheimer's disease, management strategy, and length of time in long-term care at the time when a fever developed.

Application of these results to general hospicc settings may have some limitations. The people in the study (Volicer et al., 1993) were mostly men, and their average age was lower than is typical in a general nursing facility population. Thus, additional data regarding the survival of people with advanced dementia who have diverse demographic characteristics must be collected. Inclusion of people with later-stage Alzheimer's disease in a hospice program would provide compassionate care not offered in other settings. Hospice care would be especially beneficial to the families who are struggling to keep their loved ones at home as long as possible.

CONCLUSIONS

This chapter described clinical problems faced by the caregivers of people with advanced dementia and discussed some strategies that can be used in managing the disease. The author emphasized that maintenance or improvement of the quality of life may be a more appropriate goal of care in the advanced stage of the disease than striving for survival at all costs. We should add life to days, not days to life.

REFERENCES

American Psychiatric Association. (1994). *Diagnostic and statistical manual of mental disorders* (4th ed.). Washington, DC: Author.

Applebaum, G.E., King, J.E., & Finucane, T.E. (1990). The outcome of CPR initiated in nursing homes. *Journal of the American Geriatrics Society, 38*, 197–200.

Bliwise, D.L. (1993). Sleep in normal aging and dementia. *Sleep, 16*, 40–81.

Breteler, M.M.B., Claus, J.J., Van Duijn, C.M., Launer, L.J., & Hofman, A. (1992). Epidemiology of Alzheimer's disease. *Epidemiology Reviews, 14*, 59–82.

Cohen-Mansfield, J., Werner, P., & Marx, M.S. (1989). An observational study of agitation in agitated nursing home residents. *International Journal of Psychogeriatrics, 1*(2), 153–165.

Emery, V.O., & Oxman, T.E. (1992). Update on the dementia spectrum of depression. *American Journal of Psychiatry, 149*, 305–317.

Evans, D.A., Funkenstein, H., Albert, M.S., Scherr, P.A., Cook, N.R., Chown, M.J., Hebert, L.E., Hennekens, C.H., & Taylor, J.O. (1989). Prevalence of Alzheimer's disease in a community population of older persons. *Journal of the American Medical Association, 262*, 2551–2556.

Fabiszewski, K.J., Volicer, B., & Volicer, L. (1990). Effect of antibiotic treatment on outcome of fevers in institutionalized Alzheimer patients. *Journal of the American Medical Association, 263*, 3168–3172.

Hall, G.R. (1993). Care of the patient with Alzheimer's disease living at home. *Nursing Clinics of North America, 23*, 31–46.

Henderson, C.T., Trumbore, L.S., Mobarhan, S., Benya, R., & Miles, T.P. (1992). Prolonged tube feeding in long-term care: Nutritional status and clinical outcomes. *Journal of the American College of Nutrition, 11*, 309–325.

Herz, L.R., Volicer, L., Ross, V., & Rheaume, Y. (1992). Single case study method for treatment of resistiveness in Alzheimer patients. *Hospital Communications in Psychiatry, 43*, 720–724.

Hirschowitz, B.I., & Molina, E. (1988). Anticholinergic potency of diphenhydramine (Benadryl) measured against bethanechol in the gastric fistula dog. *Journal of Pharmacology and Experimental Therapeutics, 226*, 171–173.

Hurley, A.C., Volicer, B., Mahoney, M.A., & Volicer, L. (1993). Palliative fever management in Alzheimer patients: Quality plus fiscal responsibility. *Advances in Nursing Science, 16*, 21–32.

Lazarus, L.W., Newton, N., Cohler, B., Lesser, J., & Schwein, C. (1987). Frequency and presentation of depressive symptoms in patients with primary degenerative dementia. *American Journal of Psychiatry, 144*, 41–45.

Little, J.T., Satlin, A., Sunderland, T., & Volicer, L. (1995). The sundown syndrome in severely demented patients with probable Alzheimer's disease. *Journal of Gerontology, Psychology, and Neurology, 8*, 103–106.

Reifler, B.V., Larson, E., Teri, L., & Poulsen, M. (1986). Dementia of the Alzheimer's type and depression. *Journal of the American Gerontology Society, 34*, 855–859.

Rheaume, Y., Riley, M.E., & Volicer, L. (1987). Meeting nutritional needs of Alzheimer patients who pace constantly. *Journal of Nutrition of the Elderly, 7*, 43–52.

Riley, M.E., & Volicer, L. (1990). Evaluation of a new nutritional supplement for patients with Alzheimer's disease. *Journal of the American Dietary Association, 90*, 433–435.

Satlin, A., Volicer, L., Ross, V., Herz, L., & Campbell, S. (1992). Bright light treatment of behavioral and sleep disturbances in Alzheimer's disease patients. *American Journal of Psychiatry, 149*, 1028–1032.

Swaab, D.F., Fliers, E., & Partiman, T.S. (1985). The suprachiasmatic nucleus of the human brain in relation to sex, age and senile dementia. *Brain Research, 342*, 37–44.

Vitiello, M.V., Bliwise, D.L., & Prinz, P.N. (1992). Sleep in Alzheimer's disease and the sundown syndrome. *Neurology, 42*(6, Suppl.), 83–94.

Vitiello, M.V., & Prinz, P.N. (1989). Alzheimer's disease: Sleep and sleep/wake patterns. *Clinics in Geriatric Medicine 5*(2), 289–298.

Volicer, B.J., Hurley, A., Fabiszewski, K.J., Montgomery, P., & Volicer, L. (1993). Predicting short-term survival for patients with advanced Alzheimer's disease. *Journal of the American Gerontology Society, 41*, 535–540.

Volicer, L., Rheaume, Y., Riley, M.E., Karner, J., & Glennon, M. (1990). Discontinuation of tube feeding in patients with dementia of the Alzheimer type. *American Journal of Alzheimer's Care, 5*, 22–25.

Volicer, L., Seltzer, B., Rheaume, Y., Fabiszewski, K., Herz, L., Shapiro, R., & Innis, P. (1987). Progression of Alzheimer-type dementia in institutionalized patients: A cross-sectional study. *Journal of Applied Gerontology, 6*, 83–94.

Volicer, L., Seltzer, B., Rheaume, Y., Karner, J., Glennon, M., Riley, M.E., & Crino, P.B. (1989). Eating difficulties in patients with probable dementia of the Alzheimer type. *Journal of Gerontology, Psychology, and Neurology, 2*, 169–176.

Warden, V.J. (1989). Waste not, want not. *Geriatric Nursing, 10*, 210–211.

Wragg, R.E., & Jeste, D.V. (1989). Overview of depression and psychosis in Alzheimer's disease. *American Journal of Psychiatry, 146*, 577–587.

5

Sexuality in the Special Care Unit

Edna L. Ballard, A.C.S.W., C.M.S.W.

Safe Places

As children
Our games included safe places:
Bases where we were safe and free;
Lines that the monster intruder could not cross;
Areas off limits, out of the games;
Parents around whose legs we wrapped ourselves yelling,
"You can't get me, I'm safe here."

Now older,
I'm still looking for safe places...

Ted Bowman[1]

INTIMACY, SEXUALITY, AND THE SEARCH FOR A "SAFE PLACE"

Our need for intimacy—the giving and receiving of affection, being valued, having a "safe place" to share and relive memories and to feel unconditional regard—begins at birth and continues throughout the life

[1]From Bowman, T. (1991, Fall). *Voices: The art and science of psychotherapy.* Adapted with permission.

span. It is an essential ingredient in a person's emotional health at every age. Individuals with Alzheimer's disease and other dementias experience significant negative consequences in relationships as personality and the ability to relate to others are gradually changed by the disease. Loss of initiative, loss of impulse control, unfamiliar mood and personality behaviors, increased dependency, forgetfulness, confusion, and suspiciousness all combine to change or completely do away with those characteristics that formed the basis of earlier relationships. The individual with dementia may become demanding and self-centered, losing sensitivity or awareness of the needs, rights, and wishes of others. For the caregiver, these changes can cause fear, anger, confusion, and a feeling of being trapped in a situation in which there is little hope or control. For many couples, the relationship may be affected in irreparable ways. A wife comments, "My husband is not only different but difficult. He looks the same, but he's not the same man I married. The essence of who he used to be is no longer there."

Intimacy and sexuality in people with Alzheimer's disease and related disorders are given low priority when planning for the care of these individuals. The more demented the individual, the less credence is given to the validity of sexual or intimacy needs. "What is clear is that the elderly, even the demented, have a capacity for sexual pleasure. This includes the need to touch and be touched, to feel warmth, and to share" (McCartney, Izeman, Rogers, & Cohen, 1987, p. 332). Yet, most long-term care facilities oppose overtly sexual relationships even where there is clear evidence of the partners' capacity to consent to and form the relationship. Sexual behaviors in special care units, both appropriate and inappropriate, present a response dilemma for staff. Inappropriate sexual behaviors are a problem less because of the frequency with which they occur than because of the difficulty staff have in being objective; that is, free from personal bias, attitudes, and beliefs that negatively influence their choice of intervention techniques.

As a rule, nursing and other staff have not had training or developed skills to support residents or to intervene confidently and appropriately in sexual matters (Wallace, 1992). Many respond by trying to avoid the issue, taking the position that it is not their responsibility or that, compared with other critical health issues, it indeed has low priority (Ballard & Poer, 1993). The simple expedient of separating residents and repressing or extinguishing sexual expression in residents has been and continues to be the norm. Explicit sexual or inappropriate behaviors (see Table 5.1), unlike other behavioral symptoms of Alzheimer's disease, have legal and moral implications for family and staff. The fear of legal consequences most often drives policies and practices governing sexual behavior among residents of nursing facilities. Issues of legality have not been sufficiently addressed to give staff, family, and residents clear guidelines regarding the sexual rights of residents in nursing facilities. The issue is made more

Table 5.1. Explicit sexual or inappropriate behaviors

- Fondling, hugging, or kissing strangers or others (e.g., nursing assistants)
- Masturbating in public
- Undressing or being naked in public
- Using sexually charged language
- Behaving or speaking suggestively
- Initiating or participating in sexual activity
- Making aggressive or repeated sexual overtures
- Exposing oneself during personal care tasks
- Urinating or defecating in public places

Source: Ballard & Poer (1993).

complex by religious, ethical, and personal factors. In the absence of clear, concise legal guidelines, staff must address more general issues of "maintenance of self-esteem, positive morale and interpersonal involvement in the nursing home setting" (Malatesta, 1989, p. 113). The primary concern for staff and family involves the person's capacity to consent. "This is a particularly thorny problem, because Alzheimer's capacity implies: 1) having sufficient information (memory) to evaluate and make a choice; 2) having sufficient judgment regarding the consequences of that choice; and 3) being able to decide freely of one's own volition" (Ballard & Poer, 1993, p. 40). Lichtenberg and Stizepek (1990) have developed a model for professionals to use in assessing the person's capacity to consent in sexual matters. The model includes the following guidelines:

1. Person's awareness of the relationship
   - Is the person aware of who is initiating sexual contact?
   - Does the person believe that the other person is a spouse and thus acquiesces out of a delusional belief, or is he or she cognizant of the other's identity and intent?
   - Can the person state what level of sexual intimacy he or she would be comfortable with?
2. Person's ability to avoid exploitation
   - Is the behavior consistent with formerly held beliefs/values?
   - Does the person have the ability to say no to any uninvited sexual contact?
3. Person's awareness of potential risks
   - Does the person realize that this relationship may be time limited?
   - Can the person describe how he or she will react when the relationship ends?

McLean (1994) and others argue that to rely solely on cognitive competence as a measure of social functioning and as a basis for taking away the individual's sexual rights may be less valid than considering the individual's ability to relate to others in the present. "Human connectiveness," the ability to enjoy the moment, is an important, valid consideration. People who may have severe cognitive impairment may still retain "semantic memory"—the ability to assign meaning to activities in the present. Post (1995) describes this type of memory well:

> People with temporary or permanent dementia still express emotion and respond to kindness; they still respond to their environment with pleasure or fear; they still carry on conversations of a sort, even if what they utter is muddled and they no longer remember what was spoken just seconds ago; and they can be treated in a manner that lessens the moments of terror that must accompany the felt sense of discontinuity and fragmentation of self. (p. 144)

Reliance solely on cognitive competence dehumanizes and discriminates against people with dementia (McLean, 1994; Post, 1995). The person with dementia who is unable to advocate for him- or herself is, as a rule, denied sexual rights. This position is supported by society's view of who is the more normal and the more natural candidate for sexual activity (e.g., the young, the fertile, the beautiful, the healthy). The person who is institutionalized and dependent is viewed as being asexual and must be protected from sexual behaviors. The person with dementia who now behaves in unpredictable, bizarre, even childish ways; who is often frightened and confused; who is no longer productive and capable in ways that once gave him or her status and social approval; and who, with increasing losses, becomes more dependent on others is easily dismissed by a society that places "too great a value on rationality and memory" as a basis for deciding how and if one has a right to sexual expression (Post, 1995, p. 142).

The recent development of special care units for people with dementia has been a response to the growing consensus that special strategies are necessary for the optimum care of people with dementia. *Optimum care* involves tending to the whole person—physically, socially, and emotionally. "The whole idea of a special care unit is to develop a peer community, yet when intimate relationships develop, staff members are often aghast" (Hellen, 1995, p. 7). Expressions of affection and more overt sexual behavior may embarrass or anger staff, creating a negative attitude toward the resident and the behavior (Kay & Neelley, 1982):

> Staff's attitude often reflects the reactions society has towards people living in institutions. Repressive attitudes often occur due to a sense of responsibility to avoid scandal, to satisfy the director's expectations or the families of the institutionalized patient.(Trudel & Desjardins, 1992, p. 178)

A friendship developed in a nursing facility may provide comfort, security, and a boost to the individuals' self-esteem, which is continuously assaulted by losses associated with the disease process. These friendships can be painful to families, especially to a spouse, who may be grieving the loss of the marital relationship as a result of the disease. In this case a caregiver may need help in understanding and accepting these new friendships that sometimes seem to "replace" the marital relationship. "Nursing home friendships are not the same as pre-institutionalized friendships. They arise out of the immediacy of a regimented and restricted environment that is more intense than life outside of the nursing home" (Powers, 1991, p. 55). Additionally, individuals with dementia appear to support, understand, and accept each other's needs on a level that may not be verbalized, and through social activities they are able to offer each other respite from fear, loneliness, and isolation (Gwyther, 1985). The ideal special care unit creates for the person with dementia an environment that is safe, quiet, private, predictable, and staffed by people who are sensitive, understanding, and knowledgeable about their needs. In reality, special care units vary widely in their physical settings, programming, goals, and staff training. Whatever the culture of the individual nursing facility, issues of sexuality and plans for the care of each resident begin with preadmission attitudes, relationships, and experiences of the resident and his or her family.

TRANSITION: THE DISINTEGRATION OF FAMILIAR PATTERNS

Alzheimer's disease brings about many changes, including changes in sexual identity, interest, and behaviors. In most cases the pattern is a lessening of sexual interest and activity, but the person remains a sexual being. "Sexuality includes a range of feelings that comprise our humanity—feelings of warmth, comfort, touching, security, support, love, affection and mutuality" (Hartman, 1981, p. 11). This broader perspective of sexuality and intimacy must be appreciated and understood by health care professionals who work with families and the person with dementia, for whom the opportunities to meet sexual and emotional needs have been curtailed by illness or by placement in the nursing facility (Malatesta, 1989, p. 94). Professionals who work with families are reminded that caregivers and their spouses may have a range of feelings and ways of coping with the changes in their relationship. For some, intimacy, including physical sexual activity, continues to be important despite the partner's cognitive status:

> One of the greatest fallacies associated with dementia is the assumption that Alzheimer's and other related disorders end the need for reciprocal, intimate, and satisfying sexual activity between husband and wife. In reality, many couples faced with the interpersonal losses associated with Alzheimer's may experience an increased need for emotional and sexual reassurance and nurturance. (Hanks, 1992, p. 139)

An 80-year-old male caregiver writes the following:

> I submit that spousal sexual relations should not be affected, if anything might be given more attention, when one partner suffers the onset of memory loss. First, there is the physical pleasure, even at our advanced age. Then there is the recognition of the bond between us: "No matter what, we've got each other." (Ballard & Poer, 1993, pp. 21–22)

Alzheimer's disease has a significant and varying impact on intimacy and sexuality in a marriage (Gwyther, 1990; Kuhn, 1994). For some caregivers the demands of caring for the person with Alzheimer's disease so deplete them physically and emotionally that they have little interest or energy for sex.

Numerous other factors uniquely influence the caregiver's and person's response to the effects of Alzheimer's disease on their marital relationship. Many caregivers give up initiating or participating in sexual activity, believing their partner no longer understands or welcomes intimate behaviors (Hanks, 1992). Continued sexual relations present a quandary for other caregivers, who debate the value of warmth, affection, and security of sexual intercourse versus the potential negative effect of such behavior on an already compromised mate. These caregivers may choose to isolate and distance themselves from their mates prematurely (Hanks, 1992). The following thoughts were expressed by a North Carolina caregiver for whom sexual relations continued to be important and satisfying early in the disease but changed in nature as his wife became more impaired:

> My wife has always been affectionate to the *n*th degree. [Her] condition has deteriorated, and she seems to have [regressed] to a period in her life when she was chaste. Her response to any suggestion of intimacy is, "What would Mama say?" I have accepted the stage she is at and certainly respect what she believes and feels. I have lost a wife but found a friend. (Ballard & Poer, 1993, pp. 24–25)

Families go to extraordinary lengths to delay nursing facility placement. Loss of intimacy and control are primary barriers to making the decision—a decision often fraught with desperation, guilt, and a sense of "giving up." Some couples have been together 30, 40, or 50 years or more. Some have never been separated during their marriage. "Till death do us part" has literal as well as symbolic meaning for the caregiver who now struggles with long-term care decisions. Nursing facility placement represents the dissolution of a dream—the loss of someone to talk to, to hold, to share the everyday mundane minutia of marriage; the loss of years of bonding and nurturance of a comfortable and familiar relationship:

> For many couples it's important to be together regardless of the Alzheimer's patient's recognition of the spouse. Many spousal caregivers follow the patient to the facility, initially spending about as much time with the patient as they did at home. Gradually, these families come to trust the staff and may begin to let go. (Gwyther, 1988, p. 250)

Spouses in particular will experience a range of role adjustments. "Anytime roles within a role set are changed, stress can result, both for the individual as well as the marital unit" (Ade-Ridder & Kaplan, 1993, p. 19). In *Promises to Keep*, Katherine L. Karr (1991) suggests that the family's role is one of partnership with the nursing facility, each uniquely able to provide for the resident in ways the other cannot. Relieved of personal care tasks that may have become too great, families are now free to provide love, affection, and support based on a shared past with the person. Although this is a role uniquely suited to the family, the family may be confused about what its role should be and how to become involved in the family member's care. This new role may consist of visiting, being an advocate for the person, being responsible for extra amenities and personal care tasks not readily available in the nursing facility, and, of course, generally providing attention and affection. Families often equate relinquishing physical care with relinquishing emotional care. "Emotional responsibility for an Alzheimer's disease relative isn't relieved because one is relieved of physical care" (Gwyther, 1988, p. 250). Health care professionals can be supportive of caregivers who must now learn to share the care of the person with dementia. This new role for a spouse may also include intimacy issues that may have appeared early in the disease, such as the following:

- Finding new ways to meet the need for affection, affirmation, and love (for both the person with Alzheimer's disease and the caregiver) when the person with cognitive impairment is unable to fulfill these needs
- Learning how to accommodate the changing roles and expectations of the partner with dementia
- Dealing with pain, loss, and grief as the disease progresses and as the individual continues to change in his or her ability to relate in familiar ways
- Dealing with unfamiliar behavior patterns, including an increased or diminished sexual desire on the part of the individual with dementia

For each couple, intimacy needs will be different and will vary in importance. Fatigue, grief, and anxiety may prevent the healthy spouse from forming an objective perspective for coping with any changes in the partner. Caregivers may need help in understanding how Alzheimer's disease will affect the other person and what they can expect. They may be frightened or upset by some of the changes they see and will need reassurance that they are not alone in the situation they are experiencing. "Reframing the situation often helps the caregiver to acknowledge that accepting outside support does not diminish the strength of the marital bond nor does it negate the appropriateness of their previous reliance on each other" (Gwyther, 1990, p. 702). The question for many caregivers is how to find appropriate ways to continue that reliance with a marital partner who may no longer understand or have the ability to perform this role in an emotionally acceptable way.

The degree to which a spouse resolves these issues is relevant to nursing facility staff in understanding and responding to the needs of the resident. Just as it is considered good care practice to question the family during the preadmission interview about the resident's behavior, rituals, expectations, or needs regarding, for example, bathing (does the individual prefer a shower? tub bath? morning? night? twice a day?), it should be equally important to ask about the individual's expression of intimacy in the home. Is he or she affectionate? Were there special rituals between spouses? Are there special pet names or words that have meaning only to the individuals involved? Upon hearing certain phrases or observing certain behavior, staff may conclude that it is further evidence of dementia, whereas it holds special meaning for the person. Answers to basic questions about sexual behavior and attitudes before admission are necessary to begin planning to meet the emotional needs of the resident. "Rarely (however) is the family asked for data about their loved one's needs to give or receive expressions of intimacy" (Hellen, 1995, p. 13).

ROLE OF THE NURSING FACILITY

The neurological damage caused by dementia compromises many areas of intellectual functioning, creating a challenge for caregivers to provide an environment in which individuals feel accepted and valued for who they are, not for what they can or cannot do; an environment that focuses on remaining strengths, not deficits; and an environment that supports experiences of pleasure, friendship, and the satisfaction of a job well done. Sexuality and intimacy in the nursing facility cannot be divorced from the general care and well-being of the resident. Activities, programming, and staff intervention must be deliberate, thoughtful, and individualized to "create immediate pleasure, restore dignity, provide meaningful tasks, restore roles and enable friendships" (Mace, 1987, p. 13). The need to feel valued and able to make a contribution are strong even in individuals most impaired by dementia.

Affection and good self-esteem buffer feelings of being lost, confused, and incapable. Molly, a nursing facility resident, writes, "I walk around looking for Molly and I can't find her." Too many activities in nursing facilities diminish the self-esteem of the person with dementia (Karr, 1991). Folding laundry, for example, is a good activity for a resident if it is her laundry or if this were a satisfying task for her as a housewife. Childish activities, such as making crafts out of modeling clay or dried pasta or coloring in children's coloring books, send the message that the person with dementia is not taken seriously as an adult. These activities may provide special pleasure to some individuals when chosen by them (Mace, 1987). Well-planned activity programs that are person-centered rather than task-centered can create opportunities for the person to feel good about him- or herself—to accomplish a task and to make a contribution. They may help restore to the person with dementia a sense of dignity, a sense of identity, and a role to play, as shown in the following example:[2]

> Like many people with dementia, Miss Sarah often remembers how to perform a task that was important in her life. A former schoolteacher, she enjoys her present *job*—reading to five women at the adult day care center who also have cognitive impairment. For a brief time, this activity relieves the tendency of all these women to become agitated and to wander. On days when Miss Sarah is particularly agitated, she can be prompted to sit longer and with greater enthusiasm when the activities director reads and says to her, "You must sit here and watch me. You must make sure that I don't miss any words." The teacher in her, of course, responds. Miss Sarah also grades papers. The benefits of planning a person-specific rather than a task-specific activity, as in the case of Miss Sarah, are readily apparent. The activity drawing on her residual strengths provides a pleasurable, satisfying experience and the feeling of accomplishing a task worth doing.

To be effective, activities must be chosen to meet specific needs. Selection requires time and effort, but there are many appropriate ways to address self-esteem and identity needs, including sexual needs, in individuals with dementia: "There are opportunities for integrated activities and a chance for socially acceptable communication, warmth, and touching. . . . where staff is comfortable with sexual needs and feelings, they may be able to assist residents to manage with more appropriate behavior" (McCartney et al., 1987, p. 333). The reward for staff who conscientiously make this effort is a dramatic improvement in self-esteem and the emotional state of the resident (Post, 1995).

Close physical and emotional contact, the primary ingredients of intimacy, can be met in a number of ways. One of the most readily available is the use of therapeutic touch. Staff touch residents daily during the course of providing care in, for example, taking the resident's pulse, bathing, and feeding the resident, and assisting in range of motion exercises. However, touch is seldom used consciously for its inherent therapeutic value. The therapeutic value in touch is its ability to comfort, reassure, validate, and communicate caring to and for the resident. The therapeutic use of touch can be provided in several ways, which are especially suited to visiting family when staff cannot or will not provide it:

- *Spontaneous touch:* hugs, warm embraces, holding hands, special ways of caressing
- *Pragmatic touch:* massage; the brushing of hair; creaming and oiling of the skin, particularly the hands, arms, legs, and feet

[2]Example submitted by Susan Lambert, Activities Consultant, North Carolina Division of Aging, Raleigh. Used with permission.

- *Silent touch:* sitting in quiet acceptance of another's humanness; touching or holding hands (Karr, 1991)

Physical, occupational, and recreational therapists are all in a primary position to use touch in a deliberate, therapeutic mode to enhance the well-being of the residents for whom they care. Families who are overwhelmed with guilt and grief sometimes look to staff for ways to make the resident feel needed and loved. Families who ask, "What do I say or do when all he does is beg to go home?" can be helped to interpret and respond to such a plea. Even in the late stages of the disease, priority must be given to the emotional well-being of the person with dementia: "When dementia residents lose their ability to interact with words, they can still understand nonverbal communication—touch, facial expression, voice tone. The family visitor should hug and touch the resident during the visit, talk with the person in a pleasant voice tone, and smile. This can generally comfort the resident" (Hoffman & Platt, 1991, p. 196).

GUIDELINES FOR RESPONDING TO SEXUALLY CHARGED SITUATIONS

Staff report heightened tension and distress with explicit sexual behaviors in residents. Clearly defining the behavior is a critical first step in choosing an appropriate response. The following questions provide one framework for evaluating the behavior (Ballard, 1995; also see Table 5.2):

1. Exactly what is the person doing? Is the behavior sexual or does it merely appear to be? The person disrobing may be responding to a temperature change, uncomfortable clothing, or an incontinent incident. A hug or other inappropriate sexual behavior may be a bid for attention or affection or an effort to relieve boredom. Attending to the need for attention or affection before the unwarranted behavior occurs may help to allay feelings of confusion and the need to seek validation.
2. Does the behavior occur frequently or is it an occasional incident? Is there a pattern to the behavior?
3. When does it occur? For example, is it likely to occur during bath time, when the person may mistake the identity or intent of the caregiver, or at bedtime, when the person may be seeking the security and warmth of a sleeping partner, which may have been a lifetime pattern?
4. Are there environmental changes that affect the resident or clinical changes in the resident's condition?
5. Why is this behavior a problem? Does the person exhibit a loss of impulse control or poor judgment in choice of partner, or is there a safety issue (e.g., person masturbating in such a way as to cause injury)? Does the behavior cause a disruption in the normal activities in the nursing facility?

6. For whom is this behavior a problem? The person? Staff? Other residents? Families? Visitors?
7. Is there a risk/benefit to the behavior? Does the risk outweigh the benefit?

No single strategy exists for the complex needs of the person with dementia. However, recommended management techniques for explicit sexual behaviors (Sloane, 1993) include the following:

- Chart observations
- Distract with activities or attending behaviors
- Share your successes with others and continue to use techniques that work
- Monitor whereabouts of people warranting supervision and protection
- Report behavior to appropriate person (i.e., staff, family)
- Treat incident as an integral part of care plan, developing recommendation and strategies for care

Families should be considered resources in helping staff get to know the person with dementia and in individualizing care. They may have suggestions based on years of caring for the person at home. Also, families support creative and dignified responses to their loved one's need for affection and attention, as in the following:

> One family found their grandmother was easily comforted by an old rag doll she had had years earlier and saw to it that the doll stayed with the grandmother in her care facility. They later were disturbed to learn that state surveyors cited their grandmother's facility for "demeaning" treatment of adults, i.e., allowing her to have a toy. (Gwyther, 1988, p. 247)

As in this case families may occasionally have suggestions that do not fit the "conventional theories of good care practices" but work well for their family member. Other suggestions from families may include the following:

- Let my mother have stuffed toys—she may need something to hold close.
- Words are a stumbling block, an annoyance that gets in the way of what was once so easily expressed. A welcome smile for no reason, a friendly touch on the shoulder, or a pat on the hand takes so little time and means so much.
- Care centers can be lonely places. There is not much opportunity to be held or loved. A little hug will do wonders for my wife.
- Make her feel you are working for her alone *and you enjoy it.* (Duke Family Support Program, 1989, p. 9)

Staff can prevent, reduce, or modify many difficult behaviors by being sensitive to and supportive of the ever-changing needs of the person with

Table 5.2. Key questions to ask when responding to sexually charged situations

When is staff intervention required?
- Is this the appropriate place?
- Do both participants have the capacity to consent?
- Is there a potential for harm or injury?
- Is there a third party, such as a spouse or partner in the community who objects to the behavior?

What are the appropriate, available options for specific sexual behaviors?
- Support behavior (e.g., provision of privacy, therapeutic support, information)
- Distraction when and where the behavior is inappropriate or harmful
- Substitution (e.g., providing other ways to meet the affection, self-esteem, sexual needs of residents)

Is this the correct response for this situation?
- What objective is being met?

What are the measures of success?
- Whose needs are being met?

Alzheimer's disease. The techniques listed below are generally helpful in responding to difficult behavioral problems:

1. *Consistency.* Keep changes to a minimum. Residents respond better in an environment that is predictable, dependable, psychologically safe, and supportive. Much of the acting out and inappropriate behavior in a nursing facility results from anxiety, confusion, and fear, which may be mediated by a predictable routine.
2. *Distraction.* Caregivers can often defuse and control a situation with distracting tactics. The person who is masturbating or fidgeting with his clothes may be distracted with a lap board or a pillow (Hellen, 1995) or a fidget apron. (Fidget or activity aprons are designed to provide interest and stimulation for the person with dementia. The apron has a variety of items—buttons, zippers, rulers, compass—for the person to touch and explore. Items included should reflect the person's gender and past work history or a hobby.)
3. *Reassurance.* Cognitively impaired people need the security of feeling valued and respected. Reassurance may be provided in a gesture as simple as holding the individual's hand and talking in a soothing manner during a crisis. Special care must be taken to pay attention to the person who is most "unlovable" because of difficult behaviors, personality, or appearance. The staff's response to these undesirable characteristics may be contributing to the unwanted behaviors. Staff have an obligation to show respect and promote the total well-being of all residents. This includes meaningful activities that are planned and initiated based on the individual's functional ability and that should be an integral part of each person's care plan. This takes considerable

effort and time as well as ongoing monitoring for changes in the person's level of functioning. However, it is necessary for optimum care.

4. *Task sequencing.* Planning and executing tasks becomes increasingly difficult for people with dementia. Breaking down tasks into manageable steps allows individuals to perform at their level and to increase the chances of being successful at meaningful activities, a critical component for maintaining self-esteem.
5. *Realism about residents' abilities.* Individuals with Alzheimer's disease are dependent on their caregivers. It is the responsibility of caregivers to monitor the person's changing needs and to make appropriate care plans to meet new or different needs.
6. *Know strengths and limitations.* Caregivers have varying strengths, skills, training, and limitations in caring for people with dementia. Knowing what they are good at, where they need help, and when they need a break increases their effectiveness.

NECESSARY ATTRIBUTES OF STAFF: ADMINISTRATORS, NURSES, SOCIAL WORKERS, AND NURSING ASSISTANTS

The ideal staff of a nursing facility is competent, compassionate, and committed to optimum care of every resident, no matter how impaired. Competency begins with the skills and attitudes listed below (Ballard & Poer, 1993). The following skills and attitudes apply to all nursing facility staff, but particularly to the nursing assistant:

1. Knowledge about human sexuality, particularly as it applies to older people. This knowledge includes an awareness of prevailing stereotypes and erroneous attitudes regarding the sexuality of older or ill people.
2. Awareness of personal biases and attitudes about sexuality and how this influences the ability to help in an objective, useful way.
3. Ability to accept different social, cultural, or individual sexual preferences and ability to empathize and help the individual with dementia with concerns within the context of that person's lifestyle or sexual preference. "The friendships that spring up in nursing homes are sometimes incomprehensible to residents' families. What do these unlikely pairs have in common? Although we recognize the need for friends among children, adolescents, adults and even elderly non-institutionalized people, we downplay the need for friends among the institutionalized population" (Brown University, 1993, p. 2).
4. Acceptance of the validity and sexual nature of all human beings. Staff members are in a position to do harm when they fail to respect the sexual needs of the resident who seeks or expresses sexual interest.

5. Awareness of the importance, satisfaction, and rewards of sexuality at various life stages. Above all, staff must promote and support the right of both residents and caregivers to fulfilling and satisfying intimate relationships, albeit relationships that may be different for different people. (A satisfying intimate relationship does not necessarily include sexual intercourse.)
6. Sensitivity to the difficulty many people have in discussing or sharing information of a sexual nature. Caregivers may need encouragement to share concerns, and residents may be unable to express their concerns or needs. Time should be spent building rapport with residents, creating a private, comfortable climate for discussion.
7. Ability to use appropriate vocabulary, yet be comfortable and accepting of the descriptive language used by residents or caregivers of different cultural or educational groups to describe sexual activity. Caregivers should absolutely be certain that both they and the family members understand the meaning of the terms used, especially when providing information or instructions.
8. Awareness of the impact the institutional setting and rules and regulations have on basic human rights regarding intimate behaviors.
9. Understanding as to whether to attempt to provide education or therapy, depending upon training, experience, and inclination. Caregivers should be willing to refer to another professional or agency if they are unable to meet the resident's needs. Families should be referred to credible sources in the community.
10. Willingness to provide written information and references for families who are wrestling with unanswered questions and uncertainties in this area. Families do not always ask questions or remember or fully understand information given to them in a conference. Written information allows time for review and contemplation.
11. Ability to be candid and clear about conditions under which information may be shared with others, such as other members of the treatment team (e.g., physicians, therapists).

TRAINING: WHERE IT ALL BEGINS

Adequately trained and skilled staff can find ways to minimize confusion and excess disability and can help residents feel more secure in their roles as adults (Smith, 1995). Specific training for nursing assistants in caring for people with Alzheimer's disease is critical to providing optimum care. The typical nursing assistant spends more time with residents and provides more direct care than any other staff person, according to a report by the Office of Technology Assessment (1992)—as much as 90% of contact hours. Nursing assistants must be able to respond sensitively to a variety of sexual incidents (see Table 5.3).

Quality of care depends in large measure on nursing assistants—on their knowledge and understanding of Alzheimer's disease, their caregiv-

Table 5.3. Examples of sexual problems reported in nursing facilities

1. A cognitively competent man and his wife, who has Alzheimer's disease, were having intercourse. Other residents and staff expressed concern about the wife's capacity to consent.
2. A male resident with mild cognitive impairment fondles female residents with advanced dementia. Repeated talks have had little or no effect on his behavior. He believes he has done nothing wrong.
3. A male resident is threatened with discharge because of inappropriate sexual behavior toward a female resident. The staff's only response to his behavior was to threaten discharge.
4. Two residents, both of whom are married to people living in the community, became intimate. Their respective spouses were unaware of the relationship, and the couple was from different racial, religious, and social backgrounds.
5. A male resident with severe cognitive impairment was, according to him, "reprimanded and ridiculed" when he made inappropriate advances to a child visiting on his floor.

From Ballard, E., & Kuhn, D. (1996). *Sexual behaviors in nursing homes: Suggestions for care and management.* Manuscript in preparation; reprinted with permission.

ing skills, their patience, and their attitudes about sex and about increasingly dependent people. In the words of a nurse who spent many years working in nursing facilities and whose mother is now a nursing facility resident: "I don't think about the nurses taking care of my mom. I don't think about how clean the place is. I think about the nurse's assistants. They're the ones who have the most influence on her life now." Another caregiver comments, "It's the nurse's assistant who really determines what life is like for the person who must live in a nursing home. They can treat you like a person or like a lump in the bed." Nursing assistants must be trained to provide optimum care—care that goes beyond a clean, safe environment and ensures each person a care plan that allows the greatest potential within the limitations imposed by the disease. Training must focus on expecting the most for and from the person. Nursing assistants must look at the person not as an Alzheimer's patient but as a person with Alzheimer's disease. The distinction is subtle but important because it shows in a real, often unconscious way how staff members think about, treat, and plan for residents (Ballard & Gwyther, 1990).

One of the most important principles in training nursing assistants is to offer practical information that meets concrete, immediate needs on the job. For example, the nursing assistant wants to know 1) how do I talk with the person who is having language problems, 2) how do I help the person who paces all day, 3) how do I respond to the person who can sing all the words to "The Star Spangled Banner" but cannot remember the names of his or her spouse or children or even his or her own name, and 4) how do I respond to the person who is masturbating in the lobby.

Training should determine the question as well as the answer. For example, after training, question 4 should more appropriately be phrased, how can I help the person who is masturbating in the lobby? In the first instance, the typical response is to stop the behavior, with the underlying objective often being to satisfy staff, other residents, and/or family. The second instance suggests evaluating and choosing appropriate strategies that consider the needs of the resident.

In reality, even the most comprehensive training for nursing assistants may not include discussion or techniques for responding to the sexual needs of residents. Much of what becomes "problem behavior" results from the failure to plan and promote the total well-being of residents, including self-esteem, affection, and sexual needs. Energy is spent extinguishing unacceptable behaviors. Residents who try to meet sexual needs are often viewed as uninhibited and disruptive. "When basic needs of intimacy are met, people are much less angry, unhappy, and disgruntled and they are easier to care for" (Rankin, 1989, p. 14). Nursing assistants who have participated in training report feeling better about residents and about themselves, and they have confidence in their skills even when the strategies they use do not work. Through training, nursing assistants learn to be creative, flexible, and willing to try through trial and error what works best for a particular individual at a particular time. "By giving practitioners reliable and valid assessment tools, they will be more likely to consider carefully the sexual needs of their patients. Without them, the sexual rights of competent patients are unlikely to advance" (Lichtenberg & Stizepek, 1990, p. 120).

A variety of available materials, such as journal articles, videos that may trigger discussion, educational games, and exercises, may be used in training. Two videos useful in training staff from a family perspective are *A Thousand Tomorrows: Intimacy, Sexuality and Alzheimer's* and *The Tie That Binds: An Exploration in Sexuality and Intimacy of Alzheimer's Couples*. An educational game, "Sex and Aging: A Game of Awareness and Interaction," is particularly useful in exploring attitudes, biases, and personal beliefs. The following exercises are particularly effective and are highly recommended.

"What If . . .?"

Have available for discussion a variety of hypothetical scenarios with suggestions for response. Remind participants that each situation is different, and a blanket response will not be appropriate for every case. However, exercises that allow each participant to ask questions, explore options, and share concerns provide an opportunity to increase skills and comfort level in dealing with sexual problems.

The following example is provided by Ballard and Poer (1993, pp. 41–42).

- **Question:** *What if the resident incessantly abuses herself; that is, masturbates with a potentially harmful object?*
- **Response:** If the behavior is physically harmful, a physician should always be consulted. He or she may suggest treatment or a safer substitute object, if necessary. The behavior may be self-stimulation in response to boredom. Increased activities or distractions could minimize occurrence.

Sexual behaviors, which are inappropriate or difficult because of the context or manner in which they are expressed, must be viewed and managed with the same concern and skill used in managing other behavioral symptoms of the disease. In one nursing facility staff provided a resident with a vibrator and ensured privacy; this decreased inappropriate public behavior and lessened the chance of injury from the persistent use of unconventional objects for sexual stimulation. When prescribed by a physician, such an approach may be more acceptable to families. Moreover, the point must be made that the use of restraints may result in a different and possibly greater problem. Nursing facilities vary in policy and practice. "Official" policy may differ with what is actually practiced; for example, "I try to be humane and treat individuals the way I would want to be treated. I think most of the staff would agree."

Other "what if" scenarios include the following:

- What if a resident mistakes another resident for his or her spouse and initiates intimate contact?
- What if the resident undresses in the social area?
- What if a male resident exposes himself unnecessarily while receiving personal care from a nursing assistant?
- What if the resident seems frightened and confused and seeks constant reassurance from staff and others?

In using this exercise nursing assistants should be allowed to add their own "what if" scenarios. Providing a suggestion box where they can do this anonymously may increase response and make it easier to share sensitive questions.

Group Exercise

This training approach involves a group exercise that is useful in presenting any number of examples for discussion during training. Because it is a group experience, staff can participate fully without "taking ownership" of the problem or suggested solutions. For maximum effectiveness, choose subgroups of five to seven people. Give each subgroup two to three cards (see following example) and 7–10 minutes for discussion. The groups reassemble and report to the full group for comments and further suggestions. The facilitator or trainer must be alert to inappropriate suggestions.

Each card should read as follows: *List five or more things to do in the situation listed below. Then list five or more inappropriate responses.* (The instruction to include inappropriate responses is an equally important part of this exercise.) Participants may be forced to examine what are often repressive and nontherapeutic responses to sexual expression in residents. The tendency in many nursing facilities is to extinguish behavior without further considerations or any evaluation of whether there is a valid need and how that need could be met in a dignified, compassionate manner.

The situations covered in the exercises should consist of both current and anticipated problem areas, as in the following examples:

- Mrs. Barbet is often seen coming out of Mr. Slade's room. The staff suspects that they are intimately involved.
- Mrs. Pohanka is upset with her roommate, who "entertains" her own husband in her room. Yesterday, when Mrs. Pohanka returned to her room, the roommate and husband were engaged in intimate behavior. Mrs. Pohanka called the nurse.
- Mr. Leiland, who is in a wheelchair, often grabs at nurses and other staff, using suggestive, inappropriate language.
- Staff has grown tired and annoyed with Mrs. Sayer, who constantly calls for attention, such as saying "Come here nurse" and trying to hug everyone, including visitors.

Answers will vary with situations and participants. In some situations the answers will not be easy or clearly right or wrong; conclusions will be based on consensus after evaluating many relevant factors. The following examples are selected responses to the first situation listed.

Appropriate responses

- Evaluate both individuals' ability to consent.
- Chart behaviors and report to the appropriate people.
- Support behavior within the guidelines of facility policy.
- Respect residents' right to friendship and expression of affection.
- Ensure privacy when behavior is mutually acceptable.
- Evaluate the situation for potential injury or health problems (e.g., person falling out of bed designed for one; one person has a communicable disease, such as AIDS).

Inappropriate responses

- Stand outside the door and listen.
- Summarily separate the individuals by assigning to different units.
- Threaten the residents with discharge.
- Ignore the situation completely.
- Share information about sexual incidents with others inappropriately.

Staff report feeling more confident when they have had an opportunity to discuss potential problem areas and have received suggestions for appropriate responses or care techniques. A person's sexual rights should be considered in the context of the individual's well-being and best interests. Sexual behavior between two individuals may indeed be inappropriate, but it is important to evaluate the question with respect and understanding.

INDICATORS OF SUCCESS

The following observations indicate that a facility has adopted a considerate, respectful approach to residents' sexuality.

1. When the spouse has satisfactorily resolved the issue of how to relate to the mate in the nursing facility and has specific ways of meeting needs for affection and good self-esteem (e.g., visiting with specific goals or tasks that will promote pleasure, security, and well-being). Resolution may include a variety of responses, including emotional distancing from the situation.
2. When policy and practice support the well-being of the whole person—medical, social, emotional, and sexual. Like individuals in the larger community, residents have varying needs, interests, and abilities.
3. When staff feel comfortable and effective in choosing supports and interventions in sexual matters affecting residents. Staff should have access to ongoing training that provides assessment tools, management strategies, and pragmatic suggestions and guidelines for specific behaviors.
4. When families are accepted as partners in care with the staff and have specific roles and tasks in contributing to the overall well-being of residents.
5. When the administration of the nursing facility has a clear protocol for dealing with crises involving patient autonomy, ethical questions, patient safety, and family concerns.
6. When health procedures are based on federal regulations and good nursing standards designed to protect the health of residents.
7. When families are fully aware of nursing facility policies regarding sexual behaviors and activity among residents. Families should be informed of policy and practice in the preadmission stage. Families should also be asked to provide a sexual history detailing the needs, behaviors, and experiences of individuals during this period.
8. When families have been encouraged and instructed in "new ways of caring for a spouse that meets the social and emotional needs of both partners, without interfering with staff delivery of essential nursing care" (Ade-Ridder & Kaplan, 1993, p. 20).

9. When the primary goal of the special care program is to enhance the well-being of the resident, and the climate is one of helping the person to thrive, not just survive.
10. When the resident is viewed not as an Alzheimer's patient but as a person with Alzheimer's disease. Alzheimer's describes an aspect of the individual. It does not define the individual.

CONCLUSIONS

Sexual activity and intimacy issues in the nursing facility have been and will continue to be an integral part of life for residents. It is therefore essential for staff to create an environment that promotes and protects the total well-being of residents, however those needs might vary.

REFERENCES

A thousand tomorrows: Intimacy, sexuality and Alzheimer's (1995). [Video]. (Distributed by Terra Nova Films, 9848 S. Winchester Avenue, Chicago, IL 60643.)

Ade-Ridder, L., & Kaplan, L. (1993, October). Marriage, spousal caregiving, and a husband's move to a nursing home: A changing role for the wife? *Journal of Gerontological Nursing, 19*(10), 13–23.

Ballard, E.L. (1995). Attitude, myths and realities: Helping family and professional caregivers cope with sexuality in the Alzheimer's patient. *Sexuality and Disability, 13*(3), 255–270.

Ballard, E.L., & Gwyther, L.P. (1990). *Optimum care of the nursing home resident with Alzheimer's disease: "Giving a Little Extra."* Durham, NC: Joseph and Kathleen Bryan Alzheimer's Disease Research Center, Duke Medical Center.

Ballard, E.L., & Kuhn, D. (1996). *Sexual behaviors in nursing homes: Suggestions for care and management.* Manuscript in preparation.

Ballard, E.L., & Poer, C.M. (1993). *Sexuality and the Alzheimer's patient.* Durham, NC: Joseph and Kathleen Bryan Alzheimer's Disease Research Center, Duke University Center for the Study of Aging.

Brown University Long-Term Care Quality Letter. (1993, January 20). *The Later Years, 5*(1).

Duffy, L. (Producer). (1992). *The tie that binds: An exploration in sexuality intimacy of Alzheimer's couples.* [Video]. (Distributed by Minneapolis VA Medical Center [GRECC 11G], 1 Veterans Drive, Minneapolis, MN 56001.)

Duke Family Support Program, Duke Medical Center. (1989, October). *The Caregiver Newsletter, 9*(3).

Gwyther, L.P. (1985). *Care of Alzheimer's patients: A manual for nursing home staff.* Washington, DC: American Health Care Association and Alzheimer's Disease and Related Disorders Association.

Gwyther, L.P. (1988). Nursing home care issues. In M.K. Aronson (Ed.), *Understanding Alzheimer's disease* (pp. 238–257). New York: Charles Scribner's Sons.

Gwyther, L.P. (1990). Letting go: Separation individuation in a wife on an Alzheimer's patient. *Gerontologist, 30*(5), 698–702.

Hanks, N. (1992). The effects of Alzheimer's disease on the sexual attitudes and behaviors of married caregivers and their spouses. *Sexuality and Disability, 10,* 137–151.

Hartman, C. (1981). *Sexual expression: A manual for trainers.* New York: Human Sciences Press.

Hellen, C. (1995, January). Older adults with dementia still need intimacy. *Parent Care Advisor,* pp. 7–9.

Hellen, C.R. (1995, March/April). Intimacy: Nursing home residents issues and staff training. *American Journal of Alzheimer's Disease, 10*(2), 12–17.

Hoffman, S.B., & Platt, C.A. (1991). *Comforting the confused: Strategies for managing dementia.* New York: Springer Publishing.

Karr, K.L. (1991). *Promises to keep: The family's role in nursing care.* Buffalo, NY: Prometheus Books.

Kay, B., & Neelley, J.N. (1982). Sexuality and the aging: A review of current literature. *Sexuality and Disability, 5*(1), 38–46.

Kuhn, D. (1994, September/October). The changing face of sexual intimacy in Alzheimer's disease. *American Journal of Alzheimer's Care and Related Disorders and Research, 9*(5), 7–14.

Lichtenberg, P., & Stizepek, D. (1990). Assessments of institutionalized dementia patients' competencies to participate in intimate relationships. *Gerontologist, 30*(1), 117–120.

Mace, N.L. (1987, Spring). Principles of activities for persons with dementia. *Physical and Occupational Therapy in Geriatrics, 5*(3), 13–27.

Malatesta, V.J. (1989). Sexuality and the older adult: An overview with guidelines for the health care professional. *Journal of Women & Aging, 1*(4), 93–118.

McCartney, J.R., Izeman, H., Rogers, D., & Cohen, N. (1987). Sexuality and the institutionalized elderly. *Journal of American Geriatrics, 35*(4), 331–333.

McLean, A.H. (1994, September/October). What kind of love is this? Sexuality and the elderly in nursing homes. *Sciences, 34*(5), 36–39.

Office of Technology Assessment. (1992). *Special care units for people with Alzheimer's and other dementia* (OTA-H-543). Washington, DC: U.S. Government Printing Office.

Post, S.G. (1995, Spring). Dementia in our midst: The moral community. *Cambridge Quarterly of Healthcare Ethics, 4*(2), 142–147.

Powers, B.A. (1991). The meaning of nursing home friendships. *Advances in Nursing Science, 14*(2), 42–58.

Rankin, D.J. (1989, November). Intimacy and the elderly. *Nursing Homes, 38*(3), 10–14.

Schmall, V., Staton, M., & Weaver, D. *Sex and aging: A game of awareness and interaction.* [Board game]. (Available from Oregon State University, Extension Service, Corvallis, OR 97331.)

Sloane, P.D. (1993, October). Sexual behaviors in residents with dementia: Guidelines explain how to respond. *Contemporary Long-Term Care, 16*(10), 66.

Smith, D.B. (1995, May/June). Staffing and managing special care units for Alzheimer's patients. *Geriatric Nursing, 16*(3), 124–127.

Trudel, G., & Desjardins, G. (1992). Staff reactions toward the sexual behaviors of people living in institutional settings. *Sexuality and Disability, 10*(3), 173–188.

Wallace, M. (1992, November/December). Management of sexual relations among elderly residents of long-term care facilities. *Geriatric Nursing, 13*(6), 308–311.

6

Strategies in the Care of Veterans with Dementia

Susan G. Cooley, Ph.D., and
Marsha E. Goodwin-Beck, R.N.-C., M.A., M.S.N.

Since the mid-1970s, the U.S. Department of Veterans Affairs (VA) has pursued a set of strategies to address the needs of an expanding population of veterans with Alzheimer's disease and related dementias. These strategies, which are one part of VA's comprehensive efforts to serve an increasingly aging veteran population, include data collection for dementia program planning and development, research on a wide range of dementia-related topics, education and training programs and dissemination of educational materials for medical and associated health professional staff and students, and provision of clinical dementia services at individual VA medical facilities. VA administers the largest health care network in the United States, encompassing 173 hospitals, 389 outpatient clinics, 39 domiciliaries, 77 hospital-based home care programs, and 131 nursing homes. Development and application of these strategies within VA's extensive health care system benefit not only veterans and their families, but many others in the general community as well.

This chapter describes VA's current dementia strategies. After providing an overview of the changing demographics of the veteran population and the scope of Alzheimer's disease and related dementias in this population, the chapter provides examples of recent dementia research, education, and clinical activities within VA; describes several VA special care programs that are under evaluation; and addresses special issues of ethnic diversity among veterans with dementia and VA–community collaborative efforts.

CHANGING DEMOGRAPHICS WITHIN THE VETERAN POPULATION

VA's experience with the health care needs of an increasingly aging population predates such experience in the general health care community in the United States. Although the overall size of the veteran population is declining, the proportion of older veterans has increased dramatically over the past 20 years. In 1994 the median age of veterans was 56.7 years (U.S. Department of Veterans Affairs, 1994b). At that time, approximately 32% of the veteran population (over 8.4 million of the total 26.5 million veterans) was age 65 or older (U.S. Department of Veterans Affairs, 1994b), as compared to approximately 13% in the total U.S. population. The fastest-growing segments of the veteran population were the groups 85–89 years old, 75–79 years old, and 80–84 years old, with increases of 15%, 14%, and 12%, respectively, over the previous year (U.S. Department of Veterans Affairs, 1994b). The number of veterans age 65 years or older is expected to peak at 9.3 million in the year 2000, with World War II veterans comprising the majority of these individuals (Sorensen & Feild, 1994). A second peak of almost 9 million veterans age 65 years or older is expected to occur between the years 2010 and 2020, as a result of the aging of Vietnam War–era veterans (Sorensen & Feild, 1994). By the year 2010, 42% of the entire veteran population (an estimated 8.5 million of a total 20 million veterans) will be 65 years or older (Sorensen & Feild, 1994).

Although the vast majority of veterans are male, the number and percentage of female veterans are increasing. In 1994 4.5% (approximately 1.2 million) of the total veteran population was female (U.S. Department of Veterans Affairs, 1994b); 27.7% of all female veterans (an estimated 328,000 female veterans) were age 65 or older, representing 3.8% of the entire older veteran population (Sorensen & Feild, 1994). By the year 2010, 6.4% of all veterans (approximately 1.3 million veterans) will be female; female veterans age 65 or older (approximately 276,000 veterans) will comprise 22% of all female veterans and 3.2% of all veterans age 65 or older (Sorensen & Feild, 1994). Currently, the median age of female veterans (44.7 years) is declining, in contrast to the increasing median age of male veterans, as a result of the increasing number of younger women entering the military. If present trends continue, future cohorts of older veterans will contain even greater numbers of women.

SCOPE OF DEMENTIA IN THE VETERAN POPULATION

As a result of the increasing number of older veterans and the increased prevalence of dementia at higher ages, care for veterans with cognitive impairment has become a significant concern for VA. As the number of veterans with dementia continues to rise, it is anticipated that the number of these veterans seeking VA care may also continue to rise.

The number of veterans with severe dementia is expected to increase from an estimated 400,000 in 1990 to 600,000 in the year 2000 and then remain relatively stable through the year 2030 (U.S. Department of Veterans Affairs, 1989a). In addition to veterans with severe dementia, equal or higher numbers of veterans may have mild to moderate dementia. Because the veteran population is aging faster than the U.S. population as a whole, the number of dementia cases in veterans is expected to peak between the years 2000 and 2010, while the peak in the general population is not expected to occur until the year 2030 (U.S. Department of Veterans Affairs, 1989a).

The number of discharges from VA hospital and nursing home care units of veterans with a primary or secondary diagnosis of a dementing illness has more than doubled since the early 1980s, from 13,087 discharges in fiscal year 1983 to 34,480 discharges in fiscal year 1994 (U.S. Department of Veterans Affairs, 1983b, 1994c). The number of veterans with a primary or secondary diagnosis of a dementing illness remaining in VA hospital and nursing home care units during the annual 1-day census has also nearly doubled in the past decade, from 2,313 patients in fiscal year 1983 to 4,474 patients in fiscal year 1994 (U.S. Department of Veterans Affairs, 1983a, 1994a). The majority of the veterans with dementia identified during the 1994 1-day census were located on nursing home care units (54%) or acute or intermediate care medicine units (38%); a smaller number were located on psychiatric units (8%).

These discharge and annual census data represent conservative estimates of the number of veterans with dementia who are served in the VA health care system, because dementia diagnoses that are not a focus of treatment during the inpatient stay may not be recorded in the databases. In addition, the discharge and annual census data reflect inpatients only and do not include veterans with dementia diagnoses who were seen in VA outpatient settings (e.g., outpatient clinics, adult day health care programs). Currently, the VA database of outpatient clinic information indicates which clinics were visited and how often, but it does not identify patients' diagnostic codes. Beginning in 1996 VA plans to begin collecting diagnostic codes as well as procedure codes and provider information for every outpatient encounter. In addition, a database that combines both inpatient and ambulatory patient events in one file is scheduled for implementation in 1996. Thus, more detailed data for analysis of VA health care service utilization by veterans with dementia should be available in the future. These data should enhance VA's ongoing dementia care program planning and development.

DEMENTIA RESEARCH ACTIVITIES

In fiscal year 1994 VA's intramural research on Alzheimer's disease and related dementias encompassed over 400 active projects by nearly 250 VA primary investigators at 80 VA medical centers. These dementia research projects addressed a wide variety of topics, including risk factors, causes, diagnosis, clinical course, treatment, family issues, and systems of care for patients with Alzheimer's disease and related dementias. In fiscal year 1994 VA investigators received $4.6 million of VA funding for research on Alzheimer's disease and other dementias, as well as $19.9 million of non-VA funding for such research.

Given the importance of dementia issues to veterans as well as to the general population, 5 of VA's 16 Geriatric Research, Education and Clinical Centers (GRECCs) have designated major research foci that relate to various aspects of Alzheimer's disease and related dementias. These five GRECCs are located at the following VA medical centers: Bedford, Massachusetts (division of the Boston GRECC); Minneapolis, Minnesota; Palo Alto, California; Seattle/American Lake, Washington; and Sepulveda, California. Several other GRECCs also have investigators whose research addresses dementia issues. GRECC research on Alzheimer's disease and other dementias includes basic biomedical, applied clinical, rehabilitation, and health services studies.

For example, researchers at the Bedford GRECC are investigating possible factors in the etiology and pathogenesis of Alzheimer's disease, such as the role of amyloid (an insoluble starch-like protein that accumulates on organs and tissues and compromises their function) and the relationship between amyloid deposition and neurofibrillary tangle formation (Kowall, 1994). Preliminary work suggests that some people may accumulate beta amyloid in the brain without evidence of early neuronal degeneration; further work is needed to determine how these individuals differ from people with early-stage Alzheimer's disease. Other Bedford investigators have developed a scale with which to assess the progression of late stages of Alzheimer's disease, when most scales lose their sensitivity to detect further disease progression. By combining cognitive and functional deficits with occurrence of pathological symptoms, they developed a valid, reliable, seven-item scale that is easy to learn, does not lose its sensitivity until a person reaches a vegetative state, and may be useful for the evaluation of different treatment strategies in late-stage Alzheimer's disease (Volicer, Hurley, Lathi, & Kowall, 1994). Bedford investigators are also evaluating treatment outcomes and cost-effectiveness of special care programs with a palliative care philosophy. After a 2-year study they found that levels of observed patient discomfort and costs of medications, radiology, and laboratory procedures were lower in their special care units, as compared with traditional long-term units. However, patients with lower severity of Alzheimer's disease had a higher mortality rate in the special care program than in traditional long-term care (Volicer et al., 1994).

At the Minneapolis GRECC, a major avenue of investigation is the epidemiology of Alzheimer's disease and associated risk factors (e.g., Mortimer, 1994). Principal findings from an international collaborative study included the following: 1) family history of dementia, Parkinson's disease, and Down syndrome are associated with an increased risk of Alzheimer's disease; 2) very young and very old mothers have an increased risk of giving birth to children who will later develop Alzheimer's disease; 3) a history of head trauma increases the risk of Alzheimer's disease about 2.7 times in men, but not in women; 4) a history of hypothyroidism or major depressive disorder increases the risk of Alzheimer's disease; and 5) smoking appears to "protect" individuals from getting Alzheimer's disease.

Other investigators at this center are examining pharmacological and nonpharmacological treatment of behavioral disorders in Alzheimer's disease. For example, a multicomponent behavioral intervention including specific reinforcement and visual cueing was used to decrease the agitated speech and out-of-seat behavior of a person with Alzheimer's disease in an adapted work therapy setting (Bakke et al., 1994). Investigators are also exploring neuropsychological performance patterns among patients with Alzheimer's disease and other dementias. A reliable cognitive battery measuring specific memory and problem-solving areas has been developed for use with patients with mild to moderate dementia as well as with healthy older adults (Christensen, Multhaup, Nordstrom, & Voss, 1991a, b). In other work related to a 5-year study of predictors of Alzheimer's disease progression (Mortimer, Ebbitt, Jun, & Finch, 1992), investigators found that lower scores on verbal neuropsychological tests at the time of study entry, more aggressive behavior, and sleep disturbance during the first year of observation predicted faster cognitive decline, whereas paranoid behavior, hallucinations, and activity disturbances during the first year and the presence of extrapyramidal motor signs and lower scores on nonverbal neuropsychological tests at time of study entry predicted faster functional decline. The investigators suggested that hallucinations, which occurred independently of cognitive severity, may identify a distinct subgroup of individuals with rapid functional decline.

At the Palo Alto GRECC, a major research focus is the use of psychotherapy and psychoeducational interventions to reduce stress and depression in family caregivers of frail or cognitively impaired older adults. Standard cognitive and behavioral therapy techniques, such as increasing pleasant events, monitoring moods, identifying and challenging dysfunctional thoughts, and developing more adaptive interpretations of events, have been found effective in decreasing the anger and frustration often associated with caregiving (DeVries & Gallagher-Thompson, 1993). A novel intervention program has also been developed in which a classroom format designed to help participants manage their frustration more effectively is used to teach caregivers of people with Alzheimer's disease specific skills, including learning to relax in stressful situations and learning appropriate assertiveness with family members (Gallagher-Thompson & DeVries, 1994). Leaders' and participants' manuals for these "controlling frustration" classes are available in both English- and Spanish-language versions (Gallagher-Thompson, Arguello, Johnson, Moorehead, & Polich, 1992; Gallagher-Thompson, Rose, et al., 1992).

Major investigations at the Seattle/American Lake GRECC include examination of genetic abnormalities associated with Alzheimer's disease. In 1995 GRECC researchers linked the early-onset, familial form of Alzheimer's disease to a gene on chromosome 1 (Levy-Lahad, Wasco et al., 1995; Levy-Lahad, Wijsman et al., 1995), and in 1992 provided evidence for a familial Alzheimer's disease locus on chromosome 14 (Schellenberg et al., 1992). Other investigators (Lampe et al., 1994) have described the characteristics of the chromosome 14–linked familial form of Alzheimer's disease (including onset before age 50, early progressive language impairment, early-appearing muscle jerks and generalized seizures, generalized muscular rigidity, cortical atrophy, extensive senile plaques and neurofibrillary tangles, and prominent amyloid deposits) in contrast with features of the chromosome 21–linked familial forms of Alzheimer's disease (language function predominantly spared over the initial disease course, and muscle jerks, seizures, and generalized muscular rigidity all less prevalent). GRECC researchers also investigated new drug treatments for cognitive problems and noncognitive, behavioral symptoms (e.g., depression, agitation, psychosis) in Alzheimer's disease. In a 1994 review investigators concluded that interactions between several brain neurochemical systems may be involved in the pathophysiology of behavioral disturbances in Alzheimer's disease (Raskind & Peskind, 1994).

Researchers at the Sepulveda GRECC are studying biochemical and molecular aspects of Alzheimer's disease and are attempting to improve animal models for the disorder. Studies include examination of the nature and role of amyloid plaques and apolipoprotein E; both monkey and rodent models are used (Mufson et al., 1994; Winkler et al., 1994).

Additional information on the history and impact of the GRECC program, including other examples of dementia research findings by GRECC investigators, has been reported elsewhere (Goodwin & Morley, 1994).

In addition to the dementia research conducted at these and other GRECC sites, many dementia-related issues are examined at other VA medical facilities. For example, investigators at the Atlanta VA Medical Center are participating in neuropathology projects with the Consortium to Establish a Registry for Alzheimer's Disease to improve the clinical diagnosis and neuropathological confirmation of Alzheimer's disease and other dementias. These investigators recently reported that neuropathologists have confirmed Alzheimer's disease as the primary dementing illness in 87% of autopsies of Consortium study subjects who were clinically diagnosed with Alzheimer's disease. Despite this relatively high level of clinical diagnostic accuracy, they recommend further refinement of assessment batteries in order to facilitate distinction of non-Alzheimer's dementias from Alzheimer's disease (Gearing, Mirra, Hedreen, Sumi, Hansen, & Heyman, 1995).

At the Bronx (New York) VA Medical Center, recent areas of investigation include the relationship between age at onset of Alzheimer's disease and the risk of Alzheimer's disease in first-degree relatives. Researchers have found that people with an earlier age at onset of Alzheimer's disease are more likely to have relatives with Alzheimer's disease than are those with a later age at onset of the disease. In addition, they found that an onset age of 70 best differentiated individuals whose relatives were at higher risk from individuals whose relatives were at lower risk (Li et al., 1995). Other work involves examination of the rate of deterioration in Alzheimer's disease. Researchers at the Bronx VA have found that the rate of decline in Blessed test (test of information, memory, and concentration) scores of people with Alzheimer's disease is not related to initial score, gender, age of onset, or family history of dementia (Stern et al., 1992).

At the San Diego VA Medical Center, research projects since 1990 have included examination of the apolipoprotein E genotype in people with Alzheimer's disease. In a series of autopsied people with dementia, investigators determined that the epsilon 4 form of the apolipoprotein E gene occurred in 39.6% of the people with Alzheimer's disease and in 29.0% of people with a condition known as the Lewy body variant of Alzheimer's disease, but the form of the gene was found in only 10%–15% of controls without dementia. The results provided genetic evidence for the overlap between Alzheimer's disease and the Lewy body variant of the condition (Galasko et al., 1994). Other work involves investigation of the clinical features distinguishing Alzheimer's disease from other dementias. In a large study including groups of people with possible Alzheimer's disease, probable Alzheimer's disease, and mixed dementia, principal findings included the following:

1. Delusions and psychosis occurred in about one third of each group, most often in people with moderate dementia.
2. People with possible Alzheimer's disease were distinguished from people with probable Alzheimer's disease using the features of significantly more alcohol abuse, physical health problems, and focal motor or sensory findings.
3. The group of people with mixed dementia differed from the other groups by increased prevalence of cardiovascular disease, hypertension, stroke, transient ischemic attacks (localized tissue anemia due to

obstruction of the inflow of arterial blood), and exposure to general anesthesia and by a greater frequency of depressed mood, focal motor or sensory findings, and gait disorder.

4. All groups declined by about the same amount on cognitive and functional scales over 1 year, with neither extrapyramidal (outside the system that controls skilled movements) motor signs nor psychosis predicting a more rapid rate of decline.

Thus, they found various clinical features that helped to distinguish these types of dementia but did not predict the rate of progression (Corey-Bloom, Galasko, Hofstetter, Jackson, & Thal, 1993).

EDUCATIONAL INITIATIVES RELATED TO DEMENTIA

VA conducts the nation's largest coordinated education and training effort for health care professionals. Its mandate (from Congress) is to provide training for qualified practitioners for the VA health care system and for the nation. Each year, 100,000 students receive some or all of their clinical training in VA facilities through affiliations with more than 1,000 educational institutions.

In recognition of the expanding population of older veterans, VA has been promoting and coordinating interdisciplinary geriatric and gerontological programs in its 173 medical facilities since the late 1970s. Thus, many medical and associated health students who receive clinical experience in VA medical facilities learn to care for geriatric patients, including patients with Alzheimer's disease. VA also funds specialized geriatric training programs in numerous professional disciplines, including the Physician Fellowship Program in Geriatrics, Geriatric Psychiatry Fellowship Program, Geropsychology Postdoctoral Fellowship Program, and Interdisciplinary Team Training Program. Students are also allowed to participate in several other fellowship programs in which some participants regularly address aging-related issues, including dementia. These programs include the Psychiatry Research Training Fellowship Program, Dental Research Fellowship Program, Fellowship Program in Neurosciences and Traumatic Brain Injuries, Fellowship Program in Clinical Pharmacology, Pre-doctoral Nurse Fellowship Program, and VA–Robert Wood Johnson Clinical Scholars Program. Additional funding is available for master's-level advance-practice nurse students and associated health students from various disciplines who are assigned to GRECCs and to VA facilities with geriatric programs that are not Interdisciplinary Team Training Program or GRECC sites.

Education and training within VA extends beyond the training of students to the continuing education of staff at the medical facilities. In addition to sending employees to educational programs sponsored by professional, educational, and other organizations, VA has established its own continuing education system. This in-house activity involves programming within all the individual VA medical facilities as well as a network of continuing education field units. GRECCs also provide local, regional, and national continuing education programs for VA and non-VA health care professionals. Because many VA continuing education programs are open to the public, they are a major training resource for health care professionals in many communities.

Caring for people with Alzheimer's disease and related dementias has been a component or primary focus of a number of VA's continuing education programs. In addition to various dementia-related lectures and symposia at individual VA medical facilities each year, four of VA's recent multiyear national training programs have focused on related issues, including "Hospice," "Nursing Home Care of the Mentally Ill," "Medical Management in the Elderly," and "Long-Term Care in Psychiatric Hospitals." In 1994 and 1995 VA also produced or sponsored a number of satellite videoconference programs on Alzheimer's disease and other disorders. Taped copies of the following satellite programs were distributed to all VA libraries: *Diagnosis and Treatment of Alzheimer's Disease, Dental Care of Cognitively Impaired Older Adults: Prioritizing Service Needs, Progressive Aphasia: Overview and Case in Point*, and *Primary Care of Alzheimer's Disease: A Multidisciplinary Challenge.* These videotapes are available to individuals not associated with VA through interlibrary loans arranged by local community or university libraries.

VA has also developed and disseminated a variety of other educational materials on dementia. These materials include guidelines for the diagnosis and treatment of dementia (U.S. Department of Veterans Affairs, 1989a), which address issues of epidemiology, etiology, assessment, and management of patients with dementia, as well as caregiver and ethical issues. In addition, a series of 21 caregiver education pamphlets (U.S. Department of Veterans Affairs, 1989b) were developed and evaluated by the Minneapolis GRECC. Designed for family caregivers of people with dementia, each pamphlet addresses a different subject (e.g., the role of the caregiver, management of behavior problems, respite care) and therefore can be individualized to the person's situation over time. Copies of these materials were distributed to all VA medical center libraries.

Three videotapes concerning the management of Alzheimer's disease in home and health care settings were developed by the Bedford division of the Boston GRECC. These videotapes, entitled *Alzheimer's Disease and the Family Conference, Alzheimer's Disease: Managing the Later Stages in the Home*, and *Alzheimer's Disease: Managing the Later Stages in the Health Care Setting*, were distributed to all VA medical facility libraries in 1989. As mentioned earlier, individuals not associated with VA may access these videotapes and other materials through an interlibrary loan.

In addition, VA has purchased multiple sets of "Keys to Better Care" (Consult Services, Inc., 1990), a comprehensive instructional program for health care providers caring for individuals with Alzheimer's disease and related disorders. The program consists of 14 instructional modules (1 for management and 13 for primary caregivers) supplemented by a series of short videotapes illustrating issues related to the care of people with dementia. Sets of these training materials were distributed to VA regional libraries for use on a circulating basis throughout the VA system, and are being used extensively by VA staff.

The challenge of getting educational information about dementia to staff and families is constantly confronted by the VA system, as well as by the larger community. Dissemination of educational and training materials in limited quantities to a central location in VA medical facilities, such as the library, and availability of additional copies of materials at a national depot cannot guarantee that all clinicians will be aware of, see, and use the materials. Frequent and ongoing publicizing efforts, such as mention of the materials by VA staff at conferences and in various print media, as well as repeated dissemination of resource lists, are required to maintain awareness of the availability of these materials, particularly as staff members change over time. VA has had the advantage of being an integrated health care system with a nationwide communication system and has therefore been relatively successful in its dissemination efforts. Nevertheless, improving strategies for dissemination of information will remain a challenge.

CLINICAL ACTIVITIES RELATED TO DEMENTIA

VA aims to provide a comprehensive continuum of high-quality health care services for all eligible veterans, including those with dementia. Dementia programs and services developed at individual VA medical facilities serve as models for new programs at other VA facilities and in the general community. In addition, VA collaborates with other federal, state, and local agencies in order to share expertise, pool resources, and coordinate efforts in the development of new programs in a particular locality.

VA's program for veterans with dementia is currently decentralized throughout the network of VA health care facilities. In a 1988–1989 survey 32 VA facilities reported having inpatient dementia units, 27 reported a dementia consultation team, 33 reported outpatient dementia programs, and 8 had established dementia registries. These specialized services were concentrated in 56 (approximately 33%) VA facilities. Many facilities had more than one type of these programs. Decisions about the initiation of particular dementia services at VA facilities are made at the local level, based on factors such as the size of the patient population, relevant staff and other VA resources, and the presence of similar services in the community.

In 1991 site visits were made to 13 VA medical facilities with inpatient special care programs to collect data on dementia unit staffing, programming, and other resources. A summary report of these site visits (U.S.

Department of Veterans Affairs, 1993c) revealed considerable variety among the existing special care programs. For example, some served only people at various stages of a diagnosed dementia; others served people with dementia along with individuals in other diagnostic categories, such as psychiatric patients. The goals of the programs also varied. One key finding was the identification of three basic types of dementia units: diagnostic, behavioral management, and long-term care. Although there was overlap, these three basic types of programs differed in a number of operating characteristics. For example, along with differences in basic mission, differences were found in relative size, length of stay, clinical treatment approaches, and discharge planning. VA criteria and standards for the spectrum of specialized services are currently under development.

Because VA has the most comprehensive array of inpatient, outpatient, and extended care programs, continuity of care for patients, including those with Alzheimer's and related disorders, can be achieved more readily than in most other existing health care organizations. In addition to facilities with specialized services for people with dementia, the majority of VA medical facility staffs include the medical specialties most often concerned with Alzheimer's disease (including internal medicine, neurology, psychiatry, and geriatric medicine at several sites), the members of which work closely with an interdisciplinary team of nurses, psychologists, social workers, and other therapists. In addition, eligible veterans may use several kinds of VA treatment for continuing care as needed, including acute hospital and outpatient clinic care, hospital-based home care or adult day health care, nursing home care, hospice care, and, for the family, respite care. Current efforts by VA to provide primary care for all veterans will likely enhance the coordination of care for veterans, such as those with dementia, who require multiple services over time.

VA has in recent years encouraged the designation of psychogeriatric sections within VA nursing home care units (U.S. Department of Veterans Affairs, 1995). These self-contained sections are intended to meet the medical/functional and psychiatric/behavioral needs of residents, including those with dementia, whose behavioral disturbances make them difficult to integrate into traditional nursing home settings. Preliminary results of the 1994 survey of VA nursing homes indicate that 15 VA medical centers have physically separate psychogeriatric sections in their VA nursing home care units for the care of residents with dementia or other mental disorders.

VA has had a long-standing partnership with Veterans Homes that are established and operated by individual states with assistance from VA through a construction grant and per diem grant program. State Veterans Homes provide domiciliary and/or nursing home care to veterans and, in some states, to dependents of veterans. In 1994 the National Association of State Veterans Homes surveyed the 72 state veterans nursing homes to compile information related to special care units and programs.

Of the 58 state homes responding to the survey, 33 reported separate, dedicated units for the care of veterans with Alzheimer's disease and related dementias.

SPECIAL DEMENTIA CARE PROGRAMS UNDER EVALUATION

Palliative Care for People with Late-Stage Dementia

One of the major clinical demonstration programs at the Bedford GRECC is the Dementia Study Unit, which provides a continuum of care for veterans with Alzheimer's-type dementia and for their families. The overall program has three components:

1. A GRECC Outpatient Clinic, which provides diagnostic testing for veterans with dementia syndromes and follow-up and support for veterans diagnosed as having probable Alzheimer's disease
2. A Family Study Unit, which provides individual and group support to family members of outpatients with Alzheimer's disease, as well as respite care for the veteran
3. Inpatient Care Units, which provide care for veterans with late-stage Alzheimer's disease

The inpatient component of this program consists of three 25-bed units where veterans are included in a palliative care program in which they are assigned to one of five levels of care. Decisions on the level of care to which a veteran with dementia is assigned are reached at a meeting of the interdisciplinary team with family members. The levels of care range from comfort care only to use of all measures available to sustain life. Outcome evaluation of this approach to the care of people with late-stage dementia and specific research results are addressed in Chapter 4.

Comprehensive Center for Alzheimer's Disease and Neurodegenerative Disorders

A comprehensive Center for Alzheimer's Disease and Other Neurodegenerative Disorders was established in 1995 at the Oklahoma City VA Medical Center. The goal of the center is to develop and evaluate a rural health care model for the coordinated care of veterans with Alzheimer's disease or other degenerative neurological disorders in Oklahoma. Using an interdisciplinary case management approach, the center provides services including outpatient diagnosis, treatment, and follow-up care, as well as support for family and other caregivers of veterans with these disorders. Final pathological confirmation of diagnosis via autopsy is encouraged for family counseling, treatment program development, and epidemiological purposes. The use of telemedicine technology is being explored as a way to enhance communication among providers in distant settings. Collaborative relationships between VA and state and local community organizations will be coordinated in order to meet the community service needs of these patients and their families. Relevant staff education, training, and research activities will also be developed.

Adapted Work Therapy Program for Veterans with Dementia

The Adapted Work Therapy Program at the Minneapolis VA Medical Center is unique in the VA system and the private sector. The program was initiated in 1988 as a clinical demonstration based on the sheltered workshop concept, which has been used successfully with other individuals with disabilities (Ebbitt, Burns, & Christensen, 1989). The purpose of the program is to provide meaningful work in a supervised setting where work tasks are adapted to the worker's skill and ability levels. People who qualify for this program have mild to moderate Alzheimer's disease with mild to moderate memory loss, and they can no longer maintain the jobs they once held. The program involves 10–12 individuals who perform jobs within the hospital, such as folding towels, while earning a small amount of money for their work. In addition to providing a place for these individuals to continue earning a salary, socialization is a key part of the program. The person's participation in the program also allows respite for caregivers. Socialization has proven to decrease depression scores in both patients and caregivers. Several aspects of this program continue to be evaluated with the support of groups such as the Alzheimer's Association and veterans service organizations. More recently, the program has been modified to include lower-functioning veterans because of the progression of the disease in these participants and the need for such a program in these more advanced cases. This unique program also provides an ideal setting for research on the behavioral changes over time in people with dementia and interventions for disruptive behaviors (Bakke et al., 1994).

OTHER ISSUES

Two separate issues of importance to VA as it continues to address the care of people with Alzheimer's disease and other dementias are changes in the demographic characteristics of the veteran population and collaboration with other government and private sector groups in advancing knowledge in all aspects of Alzheimer's disease and other dementias, including improved models of care for this population group.

Ethnic Diversity Among Veterans with Dementia

Although the current cohort of older veterans includes relatively few nonwhites, younger veteran cohorts contain substantially more individuals from nonwhite racial backgrounds. Thus, the issue of racial and ethnic diversity among older veterans, including those with dementia, is expected to assume increasing importance in the future. VA administrative data for 1983–1993 show there has already been some increase in ethnic diversity among veterans with dementia served in VA hospitals and nursing homes. For example, in 1983 white veterans accounted for 83% of the total number of discharges from VA hospitals and nursing home care units of veterans with a primary or secondary diagnosis of a dementing illness (U.S. Department of Veterans Affairs, 1983b). African American, Hispanic, Asian, and Native American veterans accounted for 14%, 2%, 0.2%, and 0.2% of those discharges, respectively (U.S. Department of Veterans Affairs, 1983b). In 1993 the percentage of white veterans among such discharges had decreased to 78%, and the percentages among African American, Hispanic, Asian, and Native American veterans had increased to 17%, 3%, 0.3%, and 0.3%, respectively (U.S. Department of Veterans Affairs, 1993b). Similar changes in the VA 1-day census data have occurred since 1983. In 1983 of those veterans with a primary or secondary diagnosis of a dementing illness who were present in VA hospital or nursing home care units during the 1-day census, 91% were white (U.S. Department of Veterans Affairs, 1983a). The percentages of African American, Hispanic, Asian, and Native American veterans with dementia during the census were 6%, 1%, 0.2%, and 0%, respectively (U.S. Department of Veterans Affairs, 1983a). In 1993 the percentage of white veterans with dementia present during the 1-day census had decreased to 84%, and the figures for African American, Hispanic, and Native American veterans with dementia had increased to 14%, 2%, and 0.1%, respectively; the figure for Asian veterans with dementia did not change (U.S. Department of Veterans Affairs, 1993a).

As future cohorts of older veterans with dementia become more ethnically diverse than is currently the case, it will be increasingly important to consider implications of this demographic trend for future VA dementia program planning and staff education efforts. Additional information about racial/ethnic characteristics of the veteran population, use of VA medical care by minority veterans, and ethnic diversity among veterans with dementia has been reported elsewhere (Cooley, in press; Schwartz & Klein, 1994; Stockford, 1994).

Department of Veterans Affairs–Community Collaboration

VA's long-standing involvement in research and education and training and evaluation of clinical care models for people with Alzheimer's disease and other dementias has included collaboration with a number of other federal agencies, such as the National Institute on Aging, academic institutions, and community groups interested in this area. Two VA–community collaboration efforts are provided here as an examples.

Caregiver Support Activities VA is one of five member organizations that have begun to plan and develop a National Alliance for Caregiving (NAC), which would serve both caregivers of older people and the providers who support them. Other member organizations include the American Society on Aging; the National Association of Area Agencies on Aging; the National Council on the Aging; and NAC's founding sponsor,

Glaxo Wellcome Inc. Since officially beginning operation in the spring of 1995, NAC has invited other national aging organizations to participate as affiliates. The American Association of Retired Persons and the Older Women's League have accepted the invitation to participate as affiliate organizations. The NAC is focusing its efforts on the coordination of national programs in four functional areas: information and referral; outreach and public awareness; training and technical assistance; and research. Funding is being sought to support implementation of three major projects developed by the NAC.

Special Care Programs VA participates in the Workgroup for Research and Evaluation of Special Care Units (WRESCU). The mission of this workgroup, which was established in 1990, is to facilitate research and innovation pertaining to residential special care of persons with Alzheimer's disease or other forms of dementing illness. WRESCU's membership has expanded considerably over the years and includes over 100 senior-level professionals drawn from both the public and private sectors. In addition to the overall workgroup, a number of subcommittees have been formed in order to address specific topics of relevance to the group and to share the products of the subcommittees with the entire WRESCU membership. Since 1993 WRESCU members have met annually as a designated interest group at the Gerontological Society of America Scientific Meeting. Experts on Alzheimer's disease and special care units from VA have been active members of WRESCU and its subcommittees, sharing information regarding Alzheimer's research and innovative care models developed in the VA system for people with dementia.

CONCLUSIONS

Since the mid-1970s, VA has developed strategies to address the needs of an increasing number of veterans with dementia. It is clear that VA's leadership and broad experience in the areas of research, education, and clinical care of veterans with Alzheimer's disease and other dementias have benefitted many veterans and their families, as well as many people in the general community. VA's efforts in each of these key areas must continue, given the changing demographics of the veteran population that reveal a growing proportion of older veterans. Past and current efforts by VA have been accomplished by extensive collaboration between VA, other government agencies, academic affiliates, and community groups interested and involved in issues concerning individuals with Alzheimer's disease and their families. Through VA interaction with the general community, common goals can be pursued, efforts coordinated, and expertise and other resources shared, as each learns from the other. Continued collaboration in this area is of critical importance not only to VA but to the entire U.S. population.

REFERENCES

Bakke, B.L., Kvale, S., Burns, T., McCarten, J.R., Wilson, L., Maddox, M., & Cleary, J. (1994). Multicomponent intervention for agitated behavior in a person with Alzheimer's disease. *Journal of Applied Behavior Analysis, 27*(1), 175–176.

Christensen, K.J., Multhaup, K.S., Nordstrom, S., & Voss, K. (1991a). A cognitive battery for dementia: Development and measurement characteristics. *Psychological Assessment, 3*(2), 168–174.

Christensen, K.J., Multhaup, K.S., Nordstrom, S., & Voss, K. (1991b). A new cognitive battery for dementia: Relative severity of deficits in Alzheimer's disease. *Developmental Neuropsychology,* 7(4), 435–449.

Consult Services, Inc. (1990). *Keys to better care* [audiovisual instructional package]. Narberth, PA: Author.

Cooley, S.G. (in press). Ethnic diversity among veterans with dementia. In G. Yeo & D. Gallagher-Thompson (Eds.), *Ethnicity and the dementias.* Washington, DC: Taylor & Francis.

Corey-Bloom, J., Galasko, D., Hofstetter, C.R., Jackson, J.E., & Thal, L.J. (1993). Clinical features distinguishing large cohorts with possible AD, probable AD, and mixed dementia. *Journal of the American Geriatrics Society, 41*(1), 31–37.

DeVries, H., & Gallagher-Thompson, D. (1993). Cognitive/behavioral therapy and the angry caregiver. *Clinical Gerontologist, 13*(4), 53–57.

Ebbitt, B., Burns, T., & Christensen, R. (1989). Work therapy: Intervention for community-based Alzheimer's patients. *American Journal of Alzheimer's Care and Related Disorders and Research, 4*(5), 7–15.

Galasko, D., Saitoh, T., Xia, Y., Thal, L.J., Katzman, R., Hill, L.R., & Hansen, L. (1994). The apolipoprotein E allele epsilon 4 is overrepresented in patients with the Lewy body variant of Alzheimer's disease. *Neurology, 44*(10), 1950–1951.

Gallagher-Thompson, D., Arguello, D., Johnson, C., Moorehead, R.S., & Polich, T.M. (1992). Como controlar la frustracion: Una clase para cuidantes. Palo Alto, CA: Department of Veterans Affairs Medical Center. (Available from Alzheimer's Association, 800 San Antonio Road, Palo Alto, CA 94303.)

Gallagher-Thompson, D., & DeVries, H. (1994). "Coping with frustration" classes: Development and preliminary outcomes with women who care for relatives with dementia. *Gerontologist, 34*(4), 548–552.

Gallagher-Thompson, D., Rose, J., Florsheim, M., Jacome, P., Del Maestro, S., Peters, L., Arguello, D., Johnson, C., Moorehead, R.S., Polich, T.M., Chesney, M., & Thompson, L.W. (1992). Controlling your frustration: A class for caregivers. Palo Alto, CA: Department of Veterans Affairs Medical Center. (Available from Alzheimer's Assocation, 800 San Antonio Road, Palo Alto, CA 94303.)

Gearing, M., Mirra, S.S., Hedreen, J.C., Sumi, S.M., Hansen, L.A., & Heyman, A. (1995). The Consortium to Establish a Registry for Alzheimer's Disease (CERAD). X: Neuropathology confirmation of the clinical diagnosis of Alzheimer's disease. *Neurology, 45*(3, Pt. 1), 461–466.

Goodwin, M., & Morley, J.E. (1994). Geriatric research, education, and clinical centers. Their impact in the development of American geriatrics. *Journal of the American Geriatrics Society, 42*, 1012–1019.

Kowall, N. (1994). Beta amyloid neurotoxicity and neuronal degeneration in Alzheimer's disease. *Neurobiology of Aging, 15*(2), 257–258.

Lampe, T.H., Bird, T.D., Nochlin, D., Nemens, E., Risse, S.C., Sumi, S.M., Koerker, R., Leaird, B., Wier, M., & Raskind, M. (1994). Phenotype of chromosome 14-linked familial Alzheimer's disease in a large kindred. *Annals of Neurology, 36*, 368–378.

Levy-Lahad, E., Wasco, W., Poorkaj, P., Romano, D.M., Oshima, J., Pettingell, W.H., Yu, C., Jondro, P.D., Schmidt, S.D., Wang, K., Crowley, A.C., Fu, Y., Guennette, S.Y., Galas, D., Nemens, E., Wijsman, E.M., Bird, T.D., Schellenberg, G.D., & Tanzi, R.E. (1995). Candidate gene for the chromosome 1 familial Alzheimer's disease locus. *Science, 269*, 973–977.

Levy-Lahad, E., Wijsman, E.M., Nemens, E., Anderson, L., Goddard, K.A.B., Weber, J.L., Bird, T.D., & Schellenberg, G.D. (1995). A familial Alzheimer's disease locus on chromosome 1. *Science, 269*, 970–973.

Li, G., Silverman, J.M., Smith, C.J., Zaccario, M.L., Schmeidler, J., Mohs, R.C., & Davis, K.L. (1995). Age at onset and familial risk in Alzheimer's disease. *American Journal of Psychiatry, 152*(3), 424–430.

Mortimer, J.A. (1994). What are the risk factors for dementia? In F.A. Huppert, C. Brayne, and D.W. O'Connor (Eds.), *Dementia and normal aging* (pp. 208–229). New York: Cambridge University Press.

Mortimer, J.A., Ebbitt, B., Jun, S., & Finch, M.D. (1992). Predictors of cognitive and functional progression in patients with probable Alzheimer's disease. *Neurology, 42*, 1689–1696.

Mufson, E.J., Benzing, W.C., Cole, G.M., Wang, H., Emerich, D.F., Sladek, J.R., Jr., Morrison, J.H., & Kordower, J.H. (1994). Apolipoprotein E-immunoreactivity in aged rhesus monkey cortex: Colocalization with amyloid plaques. *Neurobiology of Aging, 15*, 621–627.

Raskind, M.A., & Peskind, E.R. (1994). Neurobiologic bases of noncognitive behavioral problems in Alzheimer's disease. *Alzheimer Disease and Associated Disorders, 8*(Suppl. 3), 54–60.

Schellenberg, G.D., Bird, T.D., Wijsman, E.M., Orr, H.T., Anderson, L., Nemens, E., White, J.A., Bonnycastle, L., Weber, J.L., Alonso, M.E., Potter, H., Heston, L.L., & Martin, G.M. (1992). Genetic linkage evidence for a familial Alzheimer's disease locus on chromosome 14. *Science, 258*, 668–671.

Schwartz, S.H., & Klein, R.E. (1994). *Characteristics of the veteran population by sex, race, and Hispanic origin: Data from the 1990 census* (VA Publication No. SR-008-94-1) [Statistical report]. Washington, DC: U.S. Department of Veterans Affairs.

Sorensen, K.A., & Feild, T.C. (1994). *Projections of the U.S. veteran population: 1990 to 2010* (VA Publication No. SB 008-94-3). [Statistical brief]. Washington, DC: U.S. Department of Veterans Affairs.

Stern, R.G., Mohs, R.C., Bierer, L.M., Silverman, J.M., Schmeidler, J., Davidson, M., & Davis, K.L. (1992). Deterioration on the Blessed test in Alzheimer's disease: Longitudinal data and their implications for clinical trials and identification of subtypes. *Psychiatry Research, 42*(2), 101–110.

Stockford, D. (1994). *Usage of VA medical care by minority veterans* (VA Publication No. SR-008-95-1) [Statistical report]. Washington, DC: U.S. Department of Veterans Affairs.

U.S. Department of Veterans Affairs. (1983a). Annual patient census, September 30, 1983 [Administrative data file].

U.S. Department of Veterans Affairs. (1983b). Patient treatment file [Administrative data file].

U.S. Department of Veterans Affairs. (1989a). *Dementia: Guidelines for diagnosis and treatment* (Rev.). (VA Publication No. IB 18-3). Washington, DC: Author.

U.S. Department of Veterans Affairs. (1989b). *Alzheimer's: A guide for families caring for persons with dementia-related diseases* (VA Publication No. IB 18-7 and Supplements 1–20). Washington, DC: Author.

U.S. Department of Veterans Affairs. (1993a). Annual patient census, September 30, 1993 [Administrative data file].

U.S. Department of Veterans Affairs. (1993b). Patient treatment file [Administrative data file].

U.S. Department of Veterans Affairs. (1993c). *Survey of dementia services phase III: Dementia special care units.* (VA Publication No. IB 18-11). Washington, DC: Author.

U.S. Department of Veterans Affairs. (1994a). Annual patient census, September 30, 1994 [Administrative data file].

U.S. Department of Veterans Affairs. (1994b). *Annual report of the Secretary of Veterans Affairs: Fiscal year 1994* (Depot Stock No. P92340). Washington, DC: Author.

U.S. Department of Veterans Affairs. (1994c). Patient treatment file [Administrative data file].

U.S. Department of Veterans Affairs. (1995). *Designation of psychogeriatric sections within nursing home care units.* (Veterans Health Administration Directive No. 10-95-028). Washington, DC: Author.

Volicer, L., Collard, A., Hurley, A., Bishop, C., Kern, D., & Karon, S. (1994). Impact of special care unit for patients with advanced Alzheimer's disease on patients' discomfort and costs. *Journal of the American Geriatrics Society, 42*(6), 597–603.

Volicer, L., Hurley, A.C., Lathi, D.C., & Kowall, N.W. (1994). Measurement of severity in advanced Alzheimer's disease. *Journal of Gerontology, 49*(5), M223–M226.

Winkler, J., Conner, D.J., Frautschy, S.A., Behl, C., Waite, J.J., Cole, G.M., & Thal, L.J. (1994). Lack of long-term effects after β-amyloid protein injections in rat brain. *Neurobiology of Aging, 15*, 601–607.

7

Family Concerns

Kathleen C. Buckwalter, Ph.D., R.N., F.A.A.N., Bonnie Wakefield, M.A., R.N., James A. Waterman, M.S.N., R.N., Geri R. Hall, M.A., R.N., Toni Tripp-Reimer, Ph.D., F.A.A.N., Linda A. Gerdner, M.A., R.N., and Jerry Gilmer, Ph.D.

Since the mid-1980s there has been a growing trend for long-term care facilities to offer specialized programming for people with Alzheimer's disease and related disorders. Special care programs vary widely between elaborate specially designed free-standing facilities staffed with highly trained employees and facilities that simply close off a wing to segregate confused residents from frail residents. It has been alleged that some special programs have been opened simply as a marketing strategy, to fill empty beds without concern for programming in order to meet the special needs of people with dementia and their families. This allegation has led to alarm among families, providers, regulatory agencies, and advocacy groups such as the Alzheimer's Association, which commissioned and supported this research. Policy makers and consumer advocates are expressing increased interest in protecting the public from these problems. How-

This study was supported by a grant from the Alzheimer's Association, and supported in part by an NIA grant (#3P20AG09682-03S1) to the Iowa Center for the Study of Rural Aged.

ever, few studies have systematically identified problems or examined the perceptions of consumers of special care. The purpose of this study was to determine consumer perceptions of problems and strengths in special care programs.

METHODS

A survey questionnaire was developed that included personal demographic data, facility data (e.g., size, auspices), and questions about the experience of families with care in special care programs. These questions were based on criteria developed by the Alzheimer's Association that reflect guidelines for quality care in special care programs (Alzheimer's Association, 1992). After pilot testing the questionnaire, a total of 26,465 questionnaires were distributed by the Alzheimer's Association to 19 Association chapters from October 1992 through January 1993. These chapters were in cities and towns chosen to reflect a diversity of population size, both urban and rural areas, and regional variations. Of the questionnaires that were mailed, 1,453 (5.5%) were returned by the designated cutoff date. Nearly two thirds of the returned surveys were considered to be unusable for purposes of this analysis because the respondent stated the family member resided in a nursing facility that did not have a special care program, a group home (e.g., board and care, assisted living) for people with Alzheimer's disease or memory loss, or a facility that fell into the category of "other" (e.g., the retirement community, home care, adult day services, veterans hospital). Findings from these settings have been analyzed and reported elsewhere (Collins, Buckwalter, Hall, & Tripp-Reimer, 1994) and provide informative comparative data. Thus, there were 511 usable surveys in which respondents stated that their family member resided in a special care unit or in a nursing facility that cares only for people with Alzheimer's disease or memory loss. The data set was then reduced to a new total of 453 surveys after removing a randomly selected 50% of the 116 Texas records (N = 58) to avoid overrepresentation of subjects from this region. Because of the large quantity of data obtained in this study, a summary of the quantitative results are presented first, followed by the qualitative data.

RESULTS OF QUANTITATIVE DATA ANALYSIS

For the quantitative sections of the family survey, data were analyzed descriptively using frequencies, measures of central tendency, and rank order. Results are presented in tables and summarized here.

Sample Demographics

The majority of family respondents were equally divided between spouses (41%) and adult children (41%). Responses were received from family members in 25 states, although most came from Texas, Pennsylvania, Indiana, and Ohio. In most cases, respondents or the resident (59%) paid for their care in the special care program; 32% were covered by Medicaid.

On average, facility size was 141 beds, and there was an average of 33 residents in the special care program. Most residents were still living in the special care program (72%) and had resided in the facility an average of just under 2 years (20.5 months). The majority (65%) had been admitted from their own home and had not been in other facilities before the current one.

Ratings of Quality

Table 7.1 lists the responses regarding descriptions of quality and expectations about care in the special care program. Family members rated the quality of care as follows: excellent (51%), good (32%), fair (11%), poor (2%), and very poor (3%). Only 35% of the family respondents indicated any concerns with the care, and 65% indicated no concerns. Respondents listed the best aspects of care as caring staff (23%), cleanliness (16%), good personal care (13%), and good food service (10%). Conversely, respondents noted the worst aspects of care as inadequate staff education (12%), poor personal care (11%), and inadequate staffing (11%). (*Note:* Only responses 10% or greater are reported here.) The vast majority (82%) felt that the care met their expectations and that the care was the same as that described to them prior to admission (85%). A large majority (78%) of family respondents indicated that the brochure, advertising, and preadmission interview accurately described the program and facility. Three fourths of the respondents felt their family member had adjusted well (32%) or extremely well (43%) to the program. An important findings was that 87% of the family members who responded to the survey indicated that they would place their loved one in the same facility.

The questionnaire included questions about the essential elements of a special care program as identified by the Alzheimer's Association (see Table 7.2). These elements included expectations both at the time of admission and during the stay in the facility. Family members indicated that the special care program provided these key components in almost every case. On admission, however, only about half (49% versus 48%) of the respondents reported that they had been interviewed by facility staff to identify care strategies and special resident needs and to learn about family dynamics. Notable exceptions included discussing how physicians and other staff were selected for the program (42%) and advice on alternatives to nursing facility placement (33%). Regarding responses to essential elements during the residents' stay in the special care program, the following were not consistently met (percentages reflect number responding "yes"): decorations and furniture designed to meet the special needs of residents with Alzheimer's disease or related disorders (67%); philosophy of care different from a "regular" nursing facility (67%); and special programming for the family (61%).

Table 7.1. Descriptions and expectations of care[a]

Question	Responses	
	No.	Percentage (%)
How would you describe the care received?		
Very poor	14	3
Poor	10	2
Fair or average	47	10
Good	143	32
Excellent	228	50
No answer	11	2
Did you have any concerns with the care?		
Yes	152	35
No	281	65
No answer	20	
What were the best aspects of the care?[b]		
Caring staff	279	23
Cleanliness of facility	189	16
Good personal care	159	13
Good food service	125	10
What were the worst aspects of the care?[b]		
Inadequate staff education	85	12
Poor personal care	78	11
Inadequate staffing	77	11
Did the care meet your expectations?		
Yes	346	82
No	47	11
Don't know	27	6
No answer	33	
Was the care same as that described before admission?		
Yes	343	85
No	63	16
No answer	47	
Did the brochure, advertising, or preadmission interview accurately describe the program and/or facility?		
Yes	330	78
No	44	10
Don't know	49	12
No answer	30	
How has your family member adjusted to the program?		
Very poorly	27	7
Poorly	26	6
Fair or average	51	12
Well	130	32
Extremely well	179	43
No answer	40	

continued

Table 7.1. *(continued)*

Question	Responses: No.	Percentage (%)
If you were to do it over again, would you place your loved one in the same facility?		
Yes	377	87
No	24	6
Don't know	32	7
No answer	20	

[a]*N* = 453.

[b]Because of qualitative nature, data were clustered; multiple or no responses possible.

Costs

Table 7.3 summarizes responses regarding the cost of care in special care programs. A total of 37% of the respondents indicated they were paying more because of a special Alzheimer's program, whereas 35% replied that there were no additional costs associated with special care. A large percentage (29%) of family respondents indicated they did not know if they were paying more for services in the special care program. However, extra costs were expected by 75% of the family members. In most cases (61%) extra costs were explained to the family by the facility's administration, and most family members (59%) felt that these costs were justified. Similarly, 62% of the family members responded that the care provided by the special care program was worth the extra costs. Most of the units/facilities (69%) accepted Medicaid reimbursement.

RESULTS OF THE QUALITATIVE DATA ANALYSIS

The qualitative database comprised nine survey questions that yielded data sufficiently rich for analysis. On the whole, responses were quite "thin" or brief, as would be expected from a mailed survey. Consequently, the data were subjected only to item and categorical (not thematic) analysis. Furthermore, items had highly variable response rates, ranging from 50% to 90%. Two research assistants were trained in data coding and analysis, reaching 95% intercoder agreement; data coding was then verified by an expert in qualitative methods. For ease of interpretation, the qualitative data, which elaborate upon quantitative items in the survey, are summarized according to question. Percentages in the following sections are based on all respondents (*N* = 453), although not everyone responded to each question.

Do (Did) You Have Any Concerns with the Care Your Relative Is Receiving (Received)?

Roughly one third (*N* = 169; 37%) of respondents provided additional information beyond a yes or no answer to this question. The concerns

Table 7.2. Responses evaluating essential elements of special care programs[a]

Question	Responses No.	Percentage (%)
At admission, did the following match your experience with the facility?		
1. Was a medical evaluation to diagnose the memory loss requested for your relative before admission?		
Yes	326	77
No	70	17
Don't know	27	6
No answer	30	
2. Did the facility discuss how physicians and other staff were selected for the program?		
Yes	179	42
No	194	45
Don't know	54	13
No answer	26	
3. Did the facility determine your relative's abilities, mental status, and emotional and social needs for participation in the program?		
Yes	332	77
No	67	16
Don't know	33	8
No answer	21	
4. Was the family interviewed, preferably in the home, to identify care strategies and special resident needs and to learn family dynamics?		
Yes	207	49
No	206	48
Don't know	14	3
No answer	26	
5. Did the facility make efforts to adapt the environment to meet your relative's needs? (For example, encouraging furniture or other items to be brought from home.)		
Yes	317	73
No	107	25
Don't know	11	3
No answer	18	
6. Prior to admission, did the facility advise the family of alternatives to nursing facility placement, such as in-home care or day services, and of an Alzheimer's support group?		
Yes	127	33
No	236	62
Don't know	21	6
No answer	69	

continued

Table 7.2. *(continued)*

Question	Responses No.	Percentage (%)
7. Did a family member receive a tour of the facility?		
Yes	409	95
No	18	4
Don't know	4	1
No answer	22	
8. In the admission interview, did the facility staff discuss the following:		
A. Admission criteria		
Yes	383	91
No	24	6
Don't know	15	4
No answer	31	
B. Discharge and transfer criteria		
Yes	291	72
No	83	21
Don't know	29	7
No answer	50	
C. Resident selection for the unit and room assignment		
Yes	307	76
No	81	20
Don't know	18	4
No answer	47	
D. Costs		
Yes	398	95
No	17	4
Don't know	6	1
No answer	32	
Was the special care program different from a nursing home in the following areas?		
1. Are the decorations and furniture different from the rest of the facility and designed to meet special needs of residents with Alzheimer's disease?		
Yes	280	67
No	101	24
Don't know	39	9
No answer	33	

continued

Table 7.2. *(continued)*

Question	Responses No.	Responses Percentage (%)
2. Are special precautions taken to ensure resident safety?		
Yes	412	96
No	10	2
Don't know	7	2
No answer	24	
3. Is there a safe area for wandering?		
Yes	408	96
No	14	3
Don't know	4	1
No answer	27	
4. Is the activity programming designed especially for people with Alzheimer's disease?		
Yes	375	88
No	24	6
Don't know	25	6
No answer	29	
5. Are the staff well trained in the care of residents with Alzheimer's disease?		
Yes	332	78
No	42	10
Don't know	54	13
No answer	25	
6. Are the staff knowledgeable about Alzheimer's disease?		
Yes	347	83
No	29	7
Don't know	44	11
No answer	33	
7. Does the staff demonstrate a good attitude toward your relative?		
Yes	408	96
No	10	2
Don't know	6	1
No answer	29	
8. Was the use of medications for mood or behavior control explained to you and did it seem appropriate?		
Yes	282	72
No	79	20
Don't know	30	8
No answer	62	

continued

Table 7.2. *(continued)*

Question	Responses No.	Responses Percentage (%)
9. Are fewer physical restraints used in the special care program?		
Yes	289	70
No	76	18
Don't know	48	12
No answer	40	
10. Does the philosophy of care seem different from that in a regular nursing facility?		
Yes	280	67
No	51	12
Don't know	89	21
No answer	33	
11. Does the facility offer special programming for the family to help them adjust to Alzheimer's disease and the special care program?		
Yes	262	61
No	107	25
Don't know	61	14
No answer	23	

[a]$N = 453$.

most frequently mentioned were in the areas of personal care (8%), nutritional care (5%), staff:resident ratio (5%), activity planning (3%), environment (3%), and abuse/neglect (3%). Typical responses included "He was automatically put into diapers when he was not incontinent," and "There was not enough stimulation or chance to walk around."

What Were the Reasons for Placement of the Family Member in a Unit Specializing in the Care of People with Alzheimer's Disease?

Over 90% of respondents answered this question ($N = 416$). The reasons given for placement in a special care program were (in order of frequency) person's characteristics (68%), special care program (47%), impact of caregiving on family (40%), and poor care in a nursing facility (19%). Among the person's characteristics identified were safety concerns (primarily wandering or becoming lost) (29%), diagnosis of Alzheimer's disease (22%), disruptive behavior (primarily aggression) (18%), diminished mental capacity (confused or disoriented) (11%), other illness (6%), and physical changes (3%). The placement decision was made by professionals (28%), family (13%), and the person with dementia (1%).

At the time of placement in the special care program, the people with dementia were living with their spouse (family members' home) (28%);

Table 7.3. Costs of care in special care programs[a]

Question	Responses No.	Responses Percentage (%)
Are you paying more for care because of a special Alzheimer's program?		
Yes	158	37
No	150	35
Don't know	125	29
No answer	20	
Are you paying extra costs that you did not expect (e.g., charges for activities, food, linens, basic supplies)?		
Yes	74	17
No	324	75
Don't know	33	8
No answer	22	
Were the extra costs explained to you by the administration?		
Yes	156	61
No	61	24
Don't know	37	15
No answer	199	
Were the extra costs justified?		
Yes	138	59
No	43	18
Don't know	53	23
No answer	219	
Was the care provided worth the extra cost?		
Yes	149	62
No	38	16
Don't know	53	22
No answer	213	
Does the unit/facility accept Medicaid?		
Yes	300	69
No	41	10
Yes	17	4
Don't know	75	17
No answer	20	

[a]$N = 453$.

living in another nursing facility (12%); living in the hospital (4%); or living alone (own home) (3%). Typical responses included "I personally took care of my wife for 9½ years and realized the time had come—for her sake and my own," and "I was no longer physically or mentally able to give her the care to which she was entitled."

What Results Do (Did) You Expect from Placing Your Family Member in the Alzheimer's Program?

Over 90% of respondents answered this question (*N* = 416). The majority of the responses to this question were positive. A total of 300 responses (66%) indicated that the families anticipated good nursing care and very few comments (1%) about fears regarding poor nursing care. Positive expectations included safety and a safe environment (23%), caring staff (10%), trained staff (8%), independence for the person with dementia (5%), adequate nutrition (9%), and satisfaction for the person with dementia (9%). Family members' expectations included responses related to their inability to continue the caregiving role (5%) and the relief of stress when the person was placed in the nursing facility (6%). Typical responses included "That she would be safe from walking away. That she would not injure a bedridden resident with her 'help' "; and "To have him live out what's left of his life with as much dignity as possible. Not only did the first place keep him tied up, but he was so full of Haldol he was unaware of anything."

Was the Care the Same as What Was Described to You Prior to Admission?

Over half of the respondents answered this question (*N* = 249). Slightly more responses indicated that the special care program was more favorable than described (36%), as compared to responses indicating the program was less favorable than described (31%); 13% of the respondents did not know how the care compared to preadmission descriptions. Most of the comments made about the discrepancies between the family's experience after admission and what they were told prior to admission were made regarding care of the person with dementia (33%). Other comments included those about the staff (16%), facility environment (17%), family issues (15%), administration (14%), placement decisions (14%), and finances (3%). Typical responses included "Brochures are always glowing. Nothing is ever as good as it is advertised. This facility was no exception." "Care has improved over the years as research finds new methods of helping the residents respond to different treatment and activities."

Are There Additional Differences from a Regular Integrated Nursing Home Not Previously Mentioned that You Have Noticed?

Of the 303 respondents (67%) who answered this question, 65% of the responses were positive, and their comments about special care programs included good facility (17%), good staff development (9%), good Alzheimer's program (8%), and good personal care (6%). Negative perceptions were less common and primarily covered concerns about the facility (4%), personal care (2%), and activities (<1%). Typical responses included "Nursing home is quite different. It is very nice, but seems to address those who can't do for themselves, more care than that required by those who just can't live alone any longer. Alzheimer's unit seems more like a mental ward for catatonic." Additionally, 20 comments indicated that the respondent either did not have experience in other nursing facilities or did not understand the question.

Have There Been Extra Costs that You Did Not Expect?

Only about one fourth of the respondents answered this question (*N* = 110), and the majority of responses to this question were concerns and comments about extra charges that were not expected. Categories of unexpected charges included personal care items (18%), medication (3%), food (4%), medical care (2%), and other general costs (*N* = 18; 4%). Fewer still (3%) indicated that the charges were unnecessary or for lost and/or broken personal items (2%). Exemplar responses included "They wanted my dad to supply Depends (diapers)."

At the Time of Admission, What Information Might Have Been More Helpful?

Over half of the respondents provided data for this question (*N* = 241). Areas of additional information requested by families were (in order of priority) admission process (33%), family interaction within the special care program (8%), services for the person with dementia (6%), staff (4%), finances (3%), placement (3%), and facility (1%). Approximately 8% of the family members stated the information provided was adequate, whereas another 9% did not know how to answer this question. Exemplar responses included "I really think they could not have prepared me any better. There were going to be effects regardless," and "More specific information about the role of the family and how feedback could be provided."

If You Were to Do it Over Again, Would You Place Your Loved One in the Same Facility?

As noted in Table 7.1, the majority of responses (87%) were positive, and family members indicated they would make the same decision. Only about one fourth of the respondents provided additional information on this question (*N* = 110). Issues noted by these respondents included care, staff, financing, facility, and the family's lack of knowledge regarding better facilities. Typical responses included "There was no alternative placement opportunity," and "I feel comfortable with what I'm seeing and feel good about the secured unit."

LIMITATIONS OF THE DATA ANALYSES

Caution should be exercised when generalizing from these results. Because of the sampling procedures employed and the selection of records for inclusion in the data set, the sample can be considered neither random nor representative of the population of all families with relatives in special care programs. In addition, there may be a bias in the family responses; that is, family members may feel guilty about placing loved ones in an institution and so need to report only positive perceptions about the program. Conversely, some families may resent having others care for their family member and consequently report only negative perceptions.

DISCUSSION

One way of looking at the relatively high levels of satisfaction with special care programs expressed by family respondents is to assume that their positive perceptions are related to their inability to differentiate and measure current care against what is thought of as "special care"; that is, families may not be sophisticated enough or knowledgeable about what constitutes special care. The majority of responses to this survey regarding the best and worst aspects of care have nothing to do with specialized care; for example, cleanliness and good food service are an expected feature of all good nursing facilities. Notably missing from this list is any mention of specialized programming and activities. One possible explanation for this absence may be that 69% of the residents had never been in a nursing facility prior to the current one; therefore, families do not have anything with which to compare the current facility.

At the same time, families are extremely vulnerable to claims of specialized care. Often families wait until a crisis emerges to make a placement decision, when they may be forced to accept any available program. This notion is supported by the findings of this study, because primary reasons for placement of the family member in a special care program were characteristics of the person with dementia, including concerns about safety (wandering), progressive disease, disruptive behavior (aggression), and confusion/disorientation. When in crisis, family members are likely to believe anything they are told and may "buy into" a particular program or facility because they do not really know what the needs of their relative are or what constitutes good care. The findings of this study indicate the decisions for placement were made most often on the recommendation of a health care professional or of other family members, rather than self-referral. This suggests that families do not feel knowledgeable or confident in making decisions and need the encouragement of formal health care providers to make placement decisions. This raises the potentially troubling possibility of family vulnerability to the influence of unscrupulous providers, particularly those targeting older adults.

Families may also need to reassure themselves that they have provided the best possible care for their loved one and that the placement choice was a good one in order to alleviate feelings of guilt and abandonment. Family members responding to this survey had definite expectations about the special care program before placement, including the anticipation of good nursing care and a safe environment. However, families confronted with a unit of people with cognitive impairment may be overwhelmed by the caregiving demands they present and develop empathy for staff caregivers, whom they believe are "doing as well as can be expected." This potential for empathy is evidenced by secondary reasons for placement found in this study; that is, the burden of caregiving for the person at home. Because of this, it is possible that families may be willing to accept less than optimal care. As long as the facility is clean and has good food, specialized programming may not be as important to the families. This notion merits further investigation. However, the data from this survey are very much in keeping with the results of other family research in special care programs (Maas & Buckwalter, 1990; Mathew, Sloane, & Kirby, 1988) that supports the notion of high levels of satisfaction with care.

IMPLICATIONS FOR NURSING HOME ADMINISTRATORS

The family provides the majority of care for the person with dementia before placement in a long-term care facility. Although admission to a special care program may signify that the family can no longer manage the person at home, the role of caregiver is often not easily relinquished. Even so, this survey and others note an overall high level of satisfaction with care provided in special care programs. However, troubling issues remain. For example, in this survey, 35% of family members indicated they had some concerns about the care provided and 13% would not place their family member in the same facility. Other concerns included a lack of special programming for families and discrepancies in preadmission information and experiences with care after admission. Often, these concerns are not voiced directly to the nursing facility administrator and staff or may be invalidated by staff who believe they know what's best for the person with dementia. Unfavorable perceptions may be expressed to one of several services, including the family care review board, the nursing facility licensing agency, the Department of Human Services, the local Alzheimer's Association chapter, state and local long-term care ombudspersons, local elected officials, and/or the press.

In order to recognize the role of the family as part of the health care team, nursing home administrators must be receptive to both positive and negative feedback from family members and use this feedback to improve the quality of care for people with dementia. Therefore, every special care program should have a process in place to measure the quality of the programming, including family perceptions of care. By routinely soliciting family perceptions of care through such instruments as satisfaction questionnaires, nursing home administrators will have a valuable source of data upon which to base improvements in the program environment. Because standard patient satisfaction surveys do not address the unique needs of the person with dementia and his or her family, adapting questions from the survey reported here could yield a wealth of information about families' perceptions of the special care program.

A comprehensive quality assessment program, of which people with dementia and their families' satisfaction is one component, should be guided by a systematic plan designed to assess critical indicators of quality. In 1993 the Joint Commission on Accreditation of Healthcare Organizations developed the Dementia Special Care Unit Protocol. The protocol comprises 435 standards taken from the *Accreditation Manual for Long Term Care* that address the needs of the individual with cognitive impairment in a special care environment (Joint Commission on Accreditation of Healthcare Organizations, 1993). The protocol was tested and found to be effective in evaluating organizational performance by both professionals and consumers (Hampel & Hastings, 1993). However, findings from the pilot test indicate that test sites consistently lacked a quality improvement program specific to their special care program. If quality improvement programs are voluntarily undertaken by program administrators, there may be less need for external regulation by government agencies.

Regulatory Efforts

Although there have been complaints about special care programs, few states have enacted rules to guide program development and practice. As of 1995 seven states (Iowa, Texas, Colorado, Washington, Tennessee, Oregon, and Kansas) have adopted regulations for these programs, and at least four others (North Carolina, Nebraska, New Jersey, and Oklahoma) are in the process of developing legislation. It appears that state regulations have a positive impact on the type and quality of services provided in special care programs. However, research is still in its infancy regarding specific criteria and the benefits of these programs. Studies to date provide conflicting results, and many experts believe that it is therefore premature to establish state regulation (Gerdner & Buckwalter, in press).

In 1991 the Alzheimer's Association adopted "Legislative Principles for Alzheimer/Dementia Care in a Residential Setting," which they maintain are really just broad guidelines designed not to encourage more legislation or regulation but to provide leadership and outline direction in facilitating innovative and creative care options for people with dementia. The Alzheimer's Association recommends full implementation of and compliance with requirements of the federal nursing home reform law (Omnibus Budget Reconciliation Act of 1987; OBRA '87) and the creation of state provisions requiring full disclosure by facilities of the special services they provide. Disclosure legislation should include provisions and resources for consumer education and training of surveyors and ombudspersons. A copy of model disclosure regulation recommended by the Alzheimer's Association was published in a report by the Alzheimer's Association (1994).

In September 1992 the U.S. Office of Technology Assessment published a comprehensive document entitled *Special Care Units for People with*

Alzheimer's and Other Dementias: Consumer Education, Research, Regulatory, and Reimbursement Issues. This report cautions that, based on analysis of the relevant provisions of OBRA '87 and other special care program regulations in effect in six states, no new special regulations should be passed at this time. The report reasons that any new regulations would be superimposed on the existing regulatory structure for nursing facilities, which is already complex and multifaceted. They also suggest that OBRA '87 provides a better framework for regulating special care programs than any special regulations that have been or could be devised at this time.

Further Research

Additional research is clearly warranted (U.S. Office of Technology Assessment, 1992). For example, clinical trials with a randomized case control design are needed to determine the effectiveness of special care programs for residents, family members, and staff, as well as to assess the impact of these programs on other residents in the facility.

A number of other outcomes of interest in special care program research were not addressed in the study reported here, but also deserve attention. These outcomes were examined by Sloane (1991) and include the following items. Special care programs should slow the decline in personal care abilities that occurs with Alzheimer's disease and related disorders, which implies that the rates of decline in activities of daily living function and perhaps even in mental status should be reduced by special care as compared to traditional nursing facility care. Also, special care programs should reduce agitation and other disruptive behaviors more effectively than other care settings. Residents should interact more with other residents and staff, and excess disability should be minimized. Certain measures of physiological function, such as fitness, mobility, and maintenance of weight, should be improved if the goals of special care programs are achieved. Residents should be comfortable, both physiologically (i.e., free from pain) and psychologically (i.e., not isolated). Both families and residents should be satisfied with the care rendered and should consider the care superior to that delivered in traditional nursing facilities.

Sloane (1991) has set forth six major research questions to be addressed that are relevant to this chapter:

1. What are the characteristics of a good special care program?
2. Does good special care produce better outcomes than more traditional nursing facility care? If so, which outcomes are better, and to what extent?
3. Does the value of special care vary depending on disease stage?
4. If special care programs are effective, what are the elements of care that create that effect?
5. Are special care programs contributing to a two-class system of care, based on ability to pay privately?

6. When are increased costs justified in care of people with Alzheimer's disease and related disorders and to what extent?

Thus, in addition to outcomes research, investigators should be encouraged to attend to legal and ethical concerns as well as cost-related issues.

Investigators have encountered a number of obstacles to research in special care programs, including the fact that special care programs vary, and there are not yet agreed upon or established standards for these programs. Sloane also noted that research on these programs is extremely complex methodologically and that appropriate measures for people with dementia are not well developed and validated. Finally, research of this nature is very costly (Sloane, 1991).

Large-scale research undertakings, such as that currently under way with the Special Care Unit Initiative sponsored by the National Institute on Aging, should provide a wealth of information to determine the effectiveness of special care programs as compared to general nursing facility environments, as well as data on families of residents and staff. Under this initiative, the National Institute on Aging has funded ten research projects throughout the United States. Each study has a unique methodological focus. However, through the cooperative agreement mechanism the investigators collaborate on such issues as standardizing a definition of special care programs, assessing residents with dementia, and evaluating outcomes. The goal of this initiative is to determine the effectiveness and outcomes of special care programs in order to improve the quality of care provided to people with dementia and their families and to assist policy makers in making informed decisions.

More research is also needed on alternatives to special care programs, such as assisted living facilities, which provide supervised care in a homelike environment, campus-type settings with individualized apartments, residential care, and nursing facility units. Research on specific design features and care methods is needed. This effort could include surveys of staff nurses to evaluate current and prospective policy for the care of people with dementia in special care programs versus integrated nursing facilities, which would yield a wealth of clinical information relevant for the development of national guidelines. Analysis of program components (e.g., what constitutes specific activities for Alzheimer's disease and related disorders at various disease levels) is needed, as is research on specific programming details, such as the use of group therapy, music, pets, and video visitation (showing videotapes of family or friends in lieu of personal visits when the family cannot visit because of geographic distance or illness) at various stages of progression of the disease. Moreover, there is a need to evaluate outcomes of programs serving culturally distinct groups and programs with a high degree of heterogeneity.

A logical next step in the research process begun with this study is to analyze the approximately 1,000 family questionnaires that were returned but were not usable in this analysis because the relative was not residing in a special care program. A study comparing family respondents whose relatives were in traditional nursing facilities, group homes, hospitals, home care, and mental health institutes with the data obtained in this study is currently under way.

Finally, more research is needed to help policy makers dealing with reimbursement issues for special care programs to determine what therapies are most effective and which populations are best served by specialized care. More research is also needed to establish standards of care for long-term care and to guide families in their efforts to find the most appropriate care for their loved one.

CONCLUSIONS

In general, family members were well satisfied with the care their loved one received and would make the same decision to place their relative in the same special care program. However, a significant percentage of respondents reported that the facility could do more, such as advising them of alternatives to nursing facility placement; discussing how physicians and other staff were selected for the program; interviewing them to identify care strategies, resident needs, and family dynamics; offering special programming for the family to help them adjust; making an effort to adapt the environment to meet the relative's needs; and differentiating decorations and furniture from the rest of the facility so that they are designed to meet the special needs of residents with Alzheimer's disease. These issues could be easily remedied and attended to by special care program administrators, particularly because most of these issues involve better communication with families. Communication could be improved through 1) orientation of family members to the facility, the special care program, and their proposed role in the partnership with institutional staff in the care of residents; 2) training of family members to participate in care planning and caregiving; and 3) formation of a family–staff partnership contract that includes the goals and approaches of resident care, as well as the type and extent of care activities that the family will provide (Maas et al., 1994). The use of family satisfaction surveys will enhance this communication.

Additional costs were not a major concern for most family members; however, for those for whom this was a concern, the vast majority of costs related to those for personal care items. Other concerns noted, but to a lesser degree, included costs for medication, food, medical care, and general expenses. Families may need more information about whether these programs cost more than traditional nursing facilities, considering that 29% of the respondents did not know if they were paying more because of a special Alzheimer's disease program. Any extra and/or "hidden" costs should always be disclosed to family members prior to admission; and in our sample, this was true only 61% of the time. Preadmission discussion and disclosure of these costs is highly recommended.

REFERENCES

Alzheimer's Association. (1992). *Guidelines for dignity: Goals of specialized Alzheimer/dementia care in residential settings.* Chicago: Author.

Alzheimer's Association. (1994). *Alzheimer special care in nursing homes: Is it really special?* Chicago: Author.

Collins, C.E., Buckwalter, K.C., Hall, G.R., & Tripp-Reimer, T. (1994). Adult foster care for persons with dementia: Family perceptions of care quality (abstract). *Gerontologist, 34*(Special issue 1), 195.

Gerdner, L.A., & Buckwalter, K.C. (in press). Review of state policies regarding special care units: Implications for family consumers and health care professionals. *American Journal of Alzheimer's Care & Related Disorders and Research.*

Hampel, M.J., & Hastings, M.M. (1993). Assessing quality in nursing home dementia special care units: A pilot test of the Joint Commission protocol. *Journal of Mental Health Administration, 20*(3), 236–246.

Joint Commission on Accreditation of Healthcare Organizations. (1993, May/June). Dementia protocol to become part of long term care survey. *Joint Commission Perspectives, 13,* pp. 5, 8.

Maas, M., & Buckwalter, K.C. (1990). *Nursing evaluation research: Alzheimer's care unit.* Rockville, MD: National Institutes of Health, National Center for Nursing Research, Grant No. R01-NR01689.

Maas, M., Buckwalter, K.C., Swanson, E., Specht, J., Tripp-Reimer, T., & Hardy, M. (1994). The caring partnership: Staff and families of persons institutionalized with Alzheimer's disease. *American Journal of Alzheimer's Care & Related Disorders and Research, 9*(6) 21–30.

Mathew, L.J., & Sloane, P.D. (1991). Care on dementia units in five states. In P.D. Sloane & L.J. Mathew (Eds.), *Dementia units in long term care* (pp. 23–50). Baltimore: The Johns Hopkins University Press.

Mathew, L.J., Sloane, P., & Kirby, M. (1988). What is different about a special care unit for dementia patients? A comparative study. *American Journal of Alzheimer's Care, 3,* 6–23.

Office of Technology Assessment. (1992). *Special care units for people with Alzheimer's and other dementias: Consumer, education, research, regulatory, and reimbursement issues* (OTA-BA-403). Washington, DC: U.S. Government Printing Office.

Sloane, P.D. (1991). *Report to the DHHS Alzheimer's disease advisory panel: Health services research issues for special care units.* Washington, DC: National Institute on Aging.

8

Interior Design/Renovation of the Special Care Unit

Lucia K. DeBauge, M.Arch., Ph.D.

Architectural and interior design decisions affect the smooth operation of a special care unit and the success of a special care program. The physical unit must be planned to look and perform well. These goals are realized when architects, interior designers, special design consultants, clients, owners, and all users of the space join in a thoughtful and cooperative effort.

The information presented in this chapter is based on site visits and personal interviews at special care units in facilities around the world since 1983 (DeBauge, 1990). These anecdotal findings are predictable in special care units for residents with Alzheimer's disease. The findings are anecdotal because facilities will not release to the public or do not record specific problems or incidents of unacceptable behavior in special care units that increase staff burden unless an incident involves injury or death. Although only one or two residents may exhibit similar behaviors in relation to the design features in a unit, these behaviors can be correlated with those in other units of similar design. For example, a few male residents with Alzheimer's disease may consistently urinate in large planters placed in corners, air conditioners mounted directly below windows in bedrooms, and closets when the toilet doors are located adjacent to the closets. Months later, when the residents are incontinent, these incidents are forgotten by staff until they are interviewed about incidents of resident behavior related to special care unit architecture and interior design features.

ARCHITECTURAL AND INTERIOR DESIGN PROGRAMMING

Architectural renovation or interior design begins with a written program, which is based on interviews, research, data gathering, and information contributed by the design consultant regarding the user's needs. In this initial stage administrative philosophies and policies specific to the unit must be agreed upon. Agreement at this stage will help avoid design complications that could result from misunderstandings over the purpose of the design. These philosophies and policies involve issues including admissions and release, levels of care, integration of residents with dementia with residents without dementia, visitation, staff training, staff shift length, restraint usage, medication dispersion, emergency protocol, tube feeding/serving of meals, bathing, and supervision and security.

During the next stage, the design process, in which decisions are made and policies are set, the central question posed is whether the unit is being designed for the residents and their psychological needs or for caregiver efficiency. In some unit designs the architectural program can be written to accommodate both residents and caregivers (e.g., wider corridors to accommodate the wandering behavior of a resident with Alzheimer's disease while the linens carts used by housekeeping are also occupying the same space). In other unit designs only one user's needs can be met. The design decision should be weighed carefully by the administrator and the special design consultant because seemingly unimportant design decisions can dramatically ameliorate or exacerbate caregiver productivity and resident behavior (DeBauge, 1990). For example, bedrooms in a triangular footprint design with a direct view from the corridor to the bed and the toilet area reduces the privacy of residents. This design may even cue other residents to sleep in one of the visible beds or to use a private toilet because they cannot find the public toilet or their own room. Room intrusion by another resident has been observed to cause problem behavior among residents, such as shouting, pushing, or hitting. From the owner's perspective, it is cost effective to supervise the toilet and the bed from the corridor without entering the room, reducing the number of staff and the supervision time required. In such a case reduced staff is more important than resident privacy and room intrusion.

Architectural and interior design programming includes the client and all users of the facility, if possible. (The client may not be the administrator. The client may be a large for-profit corporation, an investment owner who wishes to add a special care unit to the existing facility to increase profit margins.) All anticipated users of a special care unit for residents with Alzheimer's disease must include housekeeping, day and night shift, and professional and support staff. Architectural programming should also include families and residents and should consider residents' past and current behavior patterns. Easily recognized, traditional door handles reduce residents' anxiety when they operate the hardware rather than sleek, modern styles, which tend to confuse residents. Knowledge of residents' past employment may also assist in design programming. For example, a resident of an Alzheimer's care unit who had been a migrant farm worker would typically fall asleep under a tree after lunch, as he had during his working years. The state health department did not permit residents to sleep outside on the ground. Including a cushioned bench under the tree as part of the design solved the problem.

The final stage of programming is a needs and assessment report, which is developed from research, surveys, studies, inventories, interviews, and observation. If the needs of all users are not represented in the design process and programming stages, the final design of the unit may not function as intended, may reduce caregiver productivity and retention, and may increase the potential for fatigue and injury. *Poor design* (i.e., a difficult-to-use environment) is assessed when one or more user groups are left out of the needs assessment phase or when the client, who is not a user of the space, overrides the decisions of others. *Dangerous design* is assessed when, for example, the design includes an exterior wandering area that follows a sloping and naturally existing terrain. Individuals with Alzheimer's disease exhibit a slowed, shuffling gait and a lack of awareness of slope or grade changes; they may fall when walking alone. Yet Alzheimer's special care unit codes do not currently require exterior wandering areas to be uniformly level and consistent in transition to the interior unit, which is more stable and safe than transitions that are not level and consistent. The cost to level an existing sloping exterior wandering area may be considered prohibitive by the client. The administration may then adopt a restraint philosophy rather than a freedom-to-wander philosophy. The restraint philosophy requires locking the exterior wandering area except when residents are accompanied outside by a nursing assistant or family member. Thus, the purpose and function of an open, safe exterior wandering area shifts to a highly restricted area where the choice of use is dictated by staff rather than residents.

The architectural programming of the bathing/toileting space for a resident with Alzheimer's disease must also reflect the requirements of this activity. For example, a combative male resident may require bathing by two to three nursing assistants. A special design consultant can offer several design solutions with options, including fewer but larger bathing areas, where all residents can be bathed. This idea may be more cost effective, safer for all (because more nursing assistants can work at one time), and more efficient as compared with smaller, more private bathing areas for each resident room. Negative aspects of this design are the loss of privacy as residents are taken to and from the bathing areas and fatigue for staff as they carry the clothes of each resident from their private rooms. These decisions must be made at the programming stage, but it is up to the client to approve increases in square footage, which affect the budget and materials. If the designer can justify that an increase in the square footage of the bathing area may reduce potential injury or fatigue, which in turn may result in reduced staff absenteeism, the increase may be granted by the client. These examples do not necessarily indicate that the building was poorly designed. In all designs there are trade-offs that are dictated by funding, site design, and client versus user needs.

DESIGN FEATURES

The following design features illustrate how design can have an impact on residents with Alzheimer's disease and their caregivers' productivity. This is not an all-inclusive list of features, but they do demonstrate the necessity for a design consultant who is knowledgeable about Alzheimer's disease, group care behavior, and institutional interior design products and materials.

Seating

A variety of seating should be offered for residents with Alzheimer's disease. Seating should vary in height, size, shape, fabric texture, and firmness. This variety reduces the potential for pressure ulcer problems because pressure is not applied repeatedly to the same location on the body when sitting.

The number and variety of institutional fabric selections have increased and improved. Homelike textures and colors are offered in "breathable vinyl," which is impervious to moisture, acids, stains, abrasion, piling, and institutional-strength cleaning chemicals but does not have the shiny look, hard plastic feel, and stick-to-the-skin qualities of vinyl.

Sofa

In selecting a sofa for an activity area, consider a love seat that offers at least one arm for support. If the arm is extended slightly over the seat, this can be used for leverage in getting up. Also, if the sofa does not have a skirt, housekeeping is more likely to move it and clean under it rather than clean around it. Select a style that has fixed cushions, or if cushions can be rotated, make sure multiple strong hook fasteners are installed in the base and sides of the sofa seat. These fasteners prevent residents from gaining access to the zippers (to avoid shredding and eating of foam padding) or from carrying off the cushions. Do not select any button or tufted upholstered seating whose style allows for pooling of moisture or removal of buttons.

Dining Tables and Chairs

Table height must be checked using existing wheelchairs to ensure the wheelchair arms clear the table top, either below or above. If a table height is established for wheelchairs, it may be too high for individuals sitting in dining chairs. Adjustable-height pedestal dining tables and ceiling-mounted tables are available, but staff must be trained to anticipate the need to change the table height before placing food on the table or seating individuals at the table. Additionally, ceiling-mounted tables may cause confusion as a result of the cluttered view of the bar supports. Some wheelchairs allow the arms to drop down slightly while dining, and others include a tray that attaches directly to the chair. Both of these features require additional caregiver time. Unless staff are trained, these features may not be implemented.

Enough room should be provided under each table for multiple wheelchairs to be pushed under the table at the same time. In many cases one wheelchair may take up all the leg room under a table, leaving little room for other residents. If the table is to be used solely by wheelchair-bound residents, place all wheelchairs together and measure the space needed. This needed space will increase the table size dramatically. Also ensure that there is enough space to rotate the wheelchair around the table legs or center pedestal. A larger circular table may accommodate this design problem.

An administrative decision should be made regarding where wheelchair diners will sit and whether they will share tables with more ambulatory residents. Evaluate the wheelchairs currently in use in the facility and establish an acceptable height. Provide tables or attachable trays that meet an acceptable clearance height for wheelchair users.

Armless dining chair design may require a resident with Alzheimer's disease to use the table in getting into and out of the chair. For safety, the table must be stable. A stable square table has four securely attached and level legs, one on each corner, rather than a center pedestal or top-heavy adjustable design that may tilt or tip over more easily. Test tables for stability by supporting the body with the edge of the table while rising from a dining chair. All dining tables and chairs must be routinely checked for loose fittings, rough edges, and worn or torn fabric. Because most armless dining chairs are stackable, they are more susceptible to damage during routine housekeeping tasks. A variety of armless seating styles are available and if used should include cushioned backs and seats for more comfort; care in stacking should be explained to housekeeping staff in order to avoid unnecessary damage to upholstery.

All dining chairs used by residents with Alzheimer's disease should have a straight leg rather than a saber leg (one that dramatically flairs out in the back). Residents may trip or fall if the chair leg extends well past the back of the chair. If the chair is sitting on carpeting, a flat metal button glider should be industry specified for the bottom of the chair to assist in movement. These gliders should also be checked periodically, especially if chairs are stacked, because the gliders can be knocked off. The loss of these gliders can cause chairs to scar rubber or vinyl floors and snag or tear carpeting.

Dining chairs with arms should have narrow arms, with the end easily fitting into the palm of the hand. They should also be upholstered or at least have padded elbow rests to protect delicate skin and bone from resting directly on a hard surface. The arm should extend over the vertical support from the main body of the chair to offer a handgrip area for the residents to pull themselves to the edge of the seat and then push themselves directly up. The stretchers that support the chair legs should not interfere with the foot being moved slightly behind the chair leg for better body balance when rising from the chair. For larger or taller residents, the available seating space of the chair should be ample.

A small stackable armchair may inhibit larger residents from getting into and out of the chair easily. Residents may also bump chair arms with a hip or leg when sitting. A repeated bumping injury can become inflamed and ulcerated simply as a result of poor chair selection.

Space Planning for Dining Area

Flexibility must be considered in planning a dining area for residents with Alzheimer's disease. Codes or standards stating the required square footage of dining space are based on the number of beds and not on the type of seating. Residents with Alzheimer's disease may be fed in a geriatric chair, wheelchair, or a reclining lounge chair. These types of seating consume more space than does seating for ambulatory residents, and cannot interfere with emergency fire egress paths or exits. The use of larger chairs requires thoughtful space planning of the dining area in order to meet safety regulations. Carefully consider the space requirements of specific seating and the potential that all residents will dine in larger chairs. If necessary, consider offering a staggered dining time and begin to plan, design, and budget for appropriate support furniture.

Furniture from Home

If residents bring chairs or other furniture from home, inspect the furniture for safety and odors. Make sure furniture is stable and has no parts that can be removed. Inspect for chipping paint and buttons that can be eaten. Chairs may not seem to have an odor until they are used, when the air held inside dried foam is emitted. Check the chair for stability, support, and odor by sitting in it. Also check for cat or dog hair, which may cause allergic reactions in some residents.

Some residents may claim a chair or an entire sofa for a nap. Watch resident behavior carefully. To avoid having residents claim chairs, similar chairs should be brought into the area. The location of the chair may be a factor. Evaluate why the chair is important and work with residents to eliminate the problem. Considerations might include the shape and size of the chair or views from the chair.

CONFLICTING AGENDAS IN DESIGN

Problems begin when the owner and/or financial backers of the facility focus strictly on high-density/high-profit designs or state they are implementing high-tech designs for people with Alzheimer's disease. The local administrator must balance this corporate interest with the opinions of professional staff, who are interested in patient comfort and caregiver convenience.

The final special care unit design depends on three related factors: budget, square footage, and choice of materials. Materials include the type, quality, and variety of materials of the unit structure and any interior design or special features. The designer must completely control at least one of the three factors to design, remodel, or retrofit (convert existing space to another use) any building. The client usually decides which factors the designer will control. For example, if a client desires a large special care unit but has a tight budget, the quality of materials is controlled by the designer. If the budget is preset and certain materials are required as a result of a unique population or codes regarding usage, the designer controls the building size. Other factors include the building site (either existing or proposed) and client/administrative philosophy regarding the user's needs.

Some states do not offer Alzheimer's certification of a licensed nursing facility, while other states offer certification in which two segments, physical structure certification and quality of care programming, must meet specific guidelines and standards. The physical unit design is under a broader but more specific scope of codes, and locked secured units are not permitted. Some facilities address the noncertification issue by offering segregated units that are not locked but still cluster residents by disease. A locked special care unit is not required in any state.

The average construction cost of newly designed special care units for Alzheimer's disease built between 1987 and 1994 ranged from $3.7 million to $5.2 million, according to an independent survey by Senior Design of Texas in 1995. Yet most nursing home administrators are seeking ways to retrofit into a special care unit for Alzheimer's disease within a budget of $30,000 or less. Thus, a typical unit retrofit of a traditional nursing facility wing includes several minor interior changes with no structural changes.

DESIGN CONSULTATION

Often, the facility owner is not the direct user and will require education in special population design to understand why unique designs may be required for safety and supervision for units designed specifically for residents with Alzheimer's disease. Hiring a consultant to review the administrative decisions regarding special care unit designs may appear unnecessary at first. However, a qualified designer with a background in programming and designing facilities for people with Alzheimer's disease may save the owner money and increase staff productivity and resident safety. Design experience only in designing facilities for older adults is not enough. It is important to develop a behavioral and preference profile of the residents, families, professional staff, maintenance, and medical personnel who are expected to use the unit.

An experienced designer must work with the professional staff to interpret this information in order to establish the correct solutions. For example, if the majority of residents are already incontinent, then cuing residents to use the toilet is not as important as supervision. The floor plan or retrofit design might be based on a suite format, with a single toilet shared by two semiprivate rooms (i.e., four beds). This design solution reduces housekeeping hours because fewer toilet areas require less cleaning, and the square footage of two smaller toilet areas is combined into one larger space. This design increases the square footage of the single toilet area so that two or more staff members can easily toilet a potentially belligerent resident. The larger toilet area also reduces staff injuries related to back strain and fatigue and increases resident safety as a result of smoother and more easily assisted transfers to the toilet. In further renovating this space, the structural walls can be retained from the previous toilet space and converted into seating alcoves in corridors or in bedrooms for residents using geriatric chairs that require larger spaces.

In a survey of retrofitted Alzheimer's special care units with similar floor plans, professional staff noted that the residents of rooms in which the toilet door was visible were more likely to be continent than were residents of rooms in which the toilet door was hidden directly behind the bedroom entrance door (DeBauge, 1990). This finding should be considered in the room designation of residents.

Only a consultant who is experienced with interior design, environment behavior, administrative budget pressures, and professional staff requirements should attempt to review facilities for Alzheimer's special care unit design and renovation. Although a design feature may seem insignificant in a nursing facility, the feature may be very important for safety and ease of caregiving.

Familiarity with Alzheimer's disease and care is important in translating problems into design solutions. Residents experiencing delusions may become fixed on a design feature and their behavior may increase the need for supervision and maintenance. For example, exposed hinges and handles are not necessary hardware in the special care unit. These design features only draw attention to storage areas and may encourage pilfering and hoarding. A change in hinge specification noted during the architectural programming stage or painting over or removing the handles in an existing or retrofitted structure does not significantly increase the design cost. Yet the reduction of pilfering behavior of residents may allow professional staff to focus on other, more important caregiver activities.

DESIGN TO PROMOTE WAYFINDING

Innovative designs have developed many different shapes for resident rooms, with an emphasis on wayfinding. Residents may find their way to a toilet or a bed, but caregiver problems begin when the bed or toilet they find is not their own but someone else's. Families become upset when another resident (particularly of the opposite sex) is found sleeping in the family member's bed. This problem may be identified as a wayfinding problem and resolved by a variety of environmental cues such as lighting, dutch doors, traffic flow, furniture location, room color, window treatments, signage, nursing station, or room reassignment for one or both residents. Signage is important for professional staff, but if a wing has only 10 resident rooms, a room should not be numbered 204-E. A number such as 4 may be simpler for both staff and residents. The resident will not need to know that his or her room is on the second floor of the east wing of a nursing facility.

COLOR MEMORY DESIGN

The concept of "homelike" addresses the psychological needs of families during admission rather than the needs of residents. Muted patterns or pale colors are nondescript and do not assist residents in wayfinding, yet they are attractive and appeal to families.

Our earliest learning experiences typically involve simple numbers, shapes, and primary colors. Much long-term memory remains intact for people with Alzheimer's disease. Basic color memory may be used as a cue for residents with Alzheimer's disease in identifying their room (DeBauge, 1992). A room painted one basic color, such as blue, with blue bedcovers and blue miniblinds that tint the room help a resident to remember that his or her room is the blue room. A resident bedroom can be all blue and still have a homelike quality. The monochromatic (single color) color scheme initiated by Senior Design of Texas (Waco, Texas) assists residents in finding their own rooms and toilets, but requires families and professionals to be trained in the environment/behavior aspect of interior design and Alzheimer's disease. Bright, colorful rooms are encouraged, with direct sunlight falling onto chairs to welcome residents to sit in them and with highly reflective surfaces that cue residents (DeBauge, 1990) as to the location of corners and edges. Hot pink dinner plates contrast dramatically with food. Carpeting is used to reduce unwanted glare. Residents with Alzheimer's disease tend to wander less when a physical location, such as a nursing station, and a person representing authority can be seen. The nursing station should be located in a highly visible area in the unit and nursing staff should consider wearing traditional white starched uniforms, hats, and insignia for ease in identification by residents with Alzheimer's disease.

CONCLUSIONS

No perfect "recipe" exists for Alzheimer's special care unit structural design because each individual reacts differently to the environment due to race, background, culture, and regional and vernacular architecture and design (DeBauge, 1993). However, certain behaviors can be anticipated. These behaviors include pilfering from other residents, picking and eating paper or paint, hallucinating, wandering, being verbally and physically aggressive, being incontinent, inappropriately using furniture and fixtures, and elopement (attempting repeatedly to leave the unit). Administrators, owners, architects, and professionals should always rely on Alzheimer's disease specialists in the design field to review and offer new or improved products and designs.

REFERENCES

DeBauge, L.K. (1990). *Alzheimer's disease special care units: A comparative study of the retrofit design.* Doctoral dissertation, Texas A&M University, College Station.

DeBauge, L.K. (1992). Alzheimer's care unit vernacular design survey of African American and American Indian facilities. Unpublished raw data.

DeBauge, L.K. (1993). International Alzheimer's care unit post occupancy evaluations, Japan, Korea, Asia, India, and Canada. Unpublished raw data.

9

Maximizing Reimbursement for Special Care Programs

Gail Harbour, R.N.

Late in the 1980s, the Health Care Finance Administration launched a pilot project to test the efficiency of Medicare and Medicaid reimbursement to nursing facilities based on identification and accountability for the actual services provided by the specific facility. The project, slated for completion in 1996, began in Maine, South Dakota, Kansas, and Mississippi. Shortly after initiation, the Medicare project moved to New York and Texas. Over 20 states are participating in some form of case-mix reimbursement system (Romano, 1994). The case-mix system has been described as sensible and fair by some in the long-term care industry. It can also be confounding and complex. As an example, the Resource Utilization Groups, Version III, has 44 categories, each with its own weight or case-mix score. A total of 29 groups are described in the *Case-Mix Classification Workbook* (Vermont Agency of Human Services, 1991) used in Vermont. Four categories encompass Alzheimer's disease and related disorders most frequently. All four of these categories are weighted in the bottom third scores for reimbursement.

The clear intent of case-mix seems to be to provide a method of paying nursing facilities a fair rate for the care they provided to more acutely ill, medically complex residents in the hope that admissions and length of stays would be shortened in the more expensive acute care facilities.

The category information is derived directly from the Minimum Data Set Plus for Nursing Home Resident Assessment and Care Plan Screening (MDS+). Responsibility for obtaining the highest possible scores lies in the hands of caregivers, the same caregivers who are charged to help each resident to be as independent as possible. As caregivers and residents meet their goals and improve, the residents' activities of daily living (ADL) scores will decrease, moving them to a lighter-weight, lower-paying score. Caregivers capture more points in this system for feeding a resident than they do for manually cuing the resident to feed him- or herself. Anyone who has ever given direct care to a person with Alzheimer's disease knows that cuing is more time consuming.

The hierarchical groups are based on rehabilitation, diagnoses, the presence of acute problems (e.g., fever, pneumonia, dehydration), and other skills that require the intervention of licensed health care providers. These groups are further defined by the amount of assistance given in the performance of ADLs.

The hierarchical groups into which most residents with Alzheimer's disease and related disorders are placed are Impaired Cognition and Challenging Behaviors. Impaired Cognition A carries an ADL Index score of 1.41; the Challenging Behaviors A group carries an ADL Index score of 1.21. Strangely, the system reimburses at a higher rate for the care of someone who is cognitively impaired without challenging behaviors when it seems obvious that more skill and time are required for the prevention of catastrophic reactions for the person exhibiting challenging behaviors. Table 9.1 illustrates a comparison of these two categories with others that require technical care. To interpret one example, the resident with mid-stage Alzheimer's disease who is placed in the Impaired Cognition group and who requires a moderate amount of assistance with ADLs will be scored at 2.32. A resident with similar ADL needs who requires a tube feeding will be scored at 2.91. This kind of scoring shows clearly how the system is designed to reimburse for technical skill rather than the time-consuming tasks of caring for a person with cognitive deficits.

To obtain a clear picture of what these "points" mean, one must look at the translation to dollars and cents. In a hypothetical but entirely realistic example, each hundredth (0.01) of a point can equal $0.17. Each hundredth of a point is significant in capturing the maximum case-mix score (Table 9.2).

Strong advocacy from everyone, particularly professionals providing the care, may bring some relief to this problem. In the meantime, we are challenged to make the most of this plan if we are to continue to provide high-quality special care for people with dementia in nursing facilities.

The bid for the health care dollar is going to become more competitive. The challenge of maximizing case-mix scores may seem overwhelming.

Table 9.1. Maximizing reimbursement for the resident with Alzheimer's disease in a case-mix system

Group	ADL Index score	Description	Case-mix weight (score)
Impaired cognition	6–10 (B)	Stages 5–6	2.32
	4–5 (A)	Stages 4–5	1.41
Challenging behaviors	6–10 (B)	Stages 6–7	2.30
	4–5 (A)	Stages 4–5	1.21
[N.A. "Atypical" severe challenging behaviors 4.81]			
Reduced physical functioning	11–15 (D)	Late stage	2.44
	16–18 (E)	Late stage	2.89
Temporary group assignments over time			
Clinically complex	6–10 (B)	Stages 4–6	2.33
	11–16 (C)	Stages 4–6	2.79
	17–18 (D)	Late stage	3.37
Low intensity rehab	4–11 (A)	Stages 4–6	2.72
Other category scoring for comparison purposes			
(8) Other rehab categories		Scores range	2.79–7.21
(3) Extensive care (tracheostomy, suctioning, IVs)		Scores range	4.23–11.91
(3) Special care (ADL scores + specific conditions that require technical skills or skilled supervision)		Scores range	2.91–3.86

Adapted from Vermont Agency of Human Services. (1991).

Table 9.2. Hypothetical case-mix analysis

Total beds	150
Current case-mix average	2.52
Factored into nursing dollars	$45.66/day
20 Alzheimer's disease and related disorders scores improve from impaired cognition A, 1.41 to impaired cognition B, 2.32	0.91/resident
Case-mix score total (2.52 × 150)	378.00
Impact of improved scores (0.91 × 20 residents with dementia)	18.2
Adjusted case-mix total	396.2
Adjusted average for facility (396.2 ÷ 150)	2.64
Factored into nursing dollars	$47.84/day
Total facility patient days/quarter (91 days × 150 beds)	13,650 total days
Medicaid occupancy of 70% (.7 × 13,650)	9,550 Medicaid days
Increases per diem/resident ($47.82 − $45.66)	$2.18
Increase in reimbursement per quarter	$20,782.13

From Roy, J. (1995). Bennington, VT: Weston Hadden Convalescent Center.

The methods of calculating scores, the detailed accountability to justify care, and the flurry of paperwork seem designed to cause providers to feel a sense of helplessness.

Given these tools with which to work, the staff must set their goals on independence for the resident with dementia and must also document the maximum amount of care provided in a 24-hour period to capture the higher ADL Index score and to identify, in a timely manner, any change in condition that might raise the hierarchical group.

MDS+/ADL INDEX SCORE CONNECTION

The Minimum Data Set Plus for Nursing Home Resident Assessment and Care Plan Screening tool clearly defines the ADL performance scores for the staff. It is not enough for the nurse manager to have expertise with MDS+/ADL Index language. It is imperative that every caregiver use the definitions of the ADL Index score form when documenting care.

Accurate interpretation of terminology can make or break the ADL Index score. For example, it is fairly obvious to most people that the paralyzed arm of the person who has had a stroke will require weight-bearing assistance (extensive assistance) during a dressing activity. The situation becomes more complicated with the resident with cognitive impairment. When rested and focused, this resident may respond well to verbal cuing. As the day wears on, fatigue or overstimulation may occur, and this resident may be unable to interpret the messages and may require manual cuing (limited assistance) or even total care to complete a simple but essential task. It would be an injustice to provide the resident with a care plan for maximum assistance. Yet the staff must be helped to recognize that the inability to perform a task is as real for people with cognitive deficits as it is for people with physical deficits. Table 9.3 provides a sample of the relationship between the ADL performance numbers on the MDS+ and the ADL Index scores of a case-mix system. Note that the frequency with which specific support is provided is an important key in obtaining the maximum score.

Although not all ADLs are calculated in the case-mix index scores, a 24-hour monitor of all ADLs promotes individualized care in planning for maximum independence even if the resident is capable of active participation in only one small activity.

SUPPORTIVE DOCUMENTATION

One solution to surviving in this complex reimbursement environment is to provide caregivers with documentation tools that will allow and promote documentation of the maximum care given over a 24-hour period, 7 days a week.

Figure 9.1 shows a sample of such a tool. The Key column provides definitions for caregivers, assisting them to be consistent with the lan-

Table 9.3. Possible connections among facility charting, definitions from the MDS+, the MDS+ codes, and the case-mix value

Facility codes	MDS+ definition	MDS+ codes	ADL score
Independent	No help or help 1–2 times	0	1
Supervision S = Self, with set-up VC = Verbal cuing	Oversight 3+ times or same + assist 1–2 times	1	1
Limited assist LA = Limited assist MC = Manual cuing	Physical assist 3+ times or more help 1–2 times	2	3
Extensive assist 1X = Extensive assist of 1 caregiver	3 or more times weight-bearing assist or total care 7 days	3/2	4
2X = Extensive assist of 1 caregiver	As above	3/3	5
Total dependence 1X = Total care by 1 caregiver	Full staff performance for 7 days	4/2	4
2X = Total care by 2 caregivers	As above	4/3	5

Note: Exact scoring methods should be determined from the state's case-mix manual. The table is a hypothetical look at bed mobility, transfers, and toilet use. The total points of the ADLs described in individual state manuals equal the ADL index score. In addition to these activities, Vermont includes a formula for determining ADL points for eating.

Adapted from Minimum Data Set Plus for Nursing Home Resident Assessment and Care Plan Screening (MDS+) and Vermont Agency of Human Services (1991).

guage of the MDS+. The Care Plan Choices column allows space for the nurse manager, with input from the staff, to plan for individualized goals by circling the ideal choice. The ADL Care Plan calendar section is designed for the caregiver to use with initials from the Key column to show how the care was actually provided. The purpose here is to capture those late-in-the-day dependencies that are seen so often in residents with Alzheimer's disease and are related to sundowning, fatigue, and decreased sensory cuing.

In addition to the example shown, the document also includes dining, positioning in bed and chair, transferring, ambulating, and performing range of motion exercises. The form is printed on paper that is 11 × 17 inches, which provides ample space for the key initials. The caregivers' initials, resident identification, and month and year appear at the bottom on the front of the form. On the reverse side, lines for comments and caregiver signatures and space are provided to document episodes of incontinence for residents who are partially incontinent. This space is help-

KEY	CARE PLAN CHOICES *Circle one — see Key*	ADL CARE PLAN																	
			1	2	3	4	5	6	7	8	9	10	11	12	13	14	15	16	17	18
	DRESSING & BATHING	D																	
D = Days	Wash above waist S, V, LA, 1X, 1T, 2T	E																	
E = Evenings	Wash above waist S, V, LA, 1X, 1T, 2T	D																	
		E																	
N = Nights	Wash below waist S, V, LA, 1X, 1T, 2T	D																	
		E																	
S = Self-care with set-up	Dress/undress below waist S, V, LA, 1X, 1T, 2T	D																	
		E																	
LA = Limited assist. (Example: manual cuing, non-wgt. bearing)	**WEEKLY BATH/SHOWER**																		
	Type:_________Day:_________ S, V, LA, 1X, 1T, 2T	D																	
		E																	
	Special shampoo____________ Circle: S, 1T, 2T Caregiver or hairdresser	D																	
		E																	
X = Extensive Assist. caregiver provides wgt.-bearing assist. (Example: holds paralyzed limb)	**MOUTH CARE**																		
	Dentures: Upper Lower S, V, LA, X, 1T	D																	
		E																	
	Partial plate: Upper Lower S, V, LA, X, 1T	D																	
		E																	
	No teeth: Upper Lower S, V, LA, X, 1T	D																	
		E																	
1–2T Total care by caregiver	Own teeth: Upper Lower S, V, LA, X, 1T	D																	
		E																	
B = Breakfast	**SHAVE**																		
	Electric or safety razor S, V, LA, X, 1T Frequency:	D																	
		E																	
D = Dinner	**TOILETING**																		
	Bathroom, bedpan, commode, toilet Incontinent Y or N__________ S, V, LA, X, 1X, 1T, 2T ( ) Document incontinence	D																	
		E																	
		N																	

Figure 9.1. Care documentation tool on which the maximum care provided to a resident over a 24-hour, 7-day period can be recorded.

ful to the nurse manager in completing the MDS+ and in providing data for realistic toilet control programs.

When implementing a new system of documentation, it is important that the staff understand the rationale of the plan. They must be helped to understand the advantages to themselves and residents in terms of professional satisfaction and high-quality resident outcomes. They will implement this kind of change only when they understand the many potential benefits. The ADL Index scores will improve as care and the documentation of that care improve.

This documentation form creates a visual graph of the resident's improvement, decline, or maintenance of function. It isolates the specific activities in which a resident can be successful. Restorative care can be enhanced, reasonable goals can be set, and success can be experienced by the staff. This kind of success is not unusual with newly admitted residents who, after adjustment, show improvement with the support of a high-quality dementia-specific care environment.

The 31-day picture helps staff to identify declines in a timely manner, to determine the need for rehabilitation intervention, and to recognize the need for new MDS+ assessments. The sometimes mistaken assumption that all declines are related to the Alzheimer's disease process can be eliminated by an astute staff.

The licensed nursing assistants of every shift can experience a sense of empowerment as they see their documentation being used actively by other interdisciplinary team members in the care planning process. Evening and night staff can see the acknowledgment of the heavier care required, and staffing needs can be justified for their shifts. Staff members enjoy the consistency of the tool on which all ADL options are presented in the same order in each medical record.

State surveyors will see that the facility places much importance on restorative care. It is obvious that while documenting the maximum amount of support required for ADLs, resident independence is supported whenever possible.

There are many timesaving features for nurse managers. When the time comes to complete the MDS+ Quarterly or Annual Assessment, it is much easier to see permanent changes in ADLs. This assessment can provide the justification for completing a full MDS+, can provide realistic goals, and can simultaneously increase the ADL score in a timely manner.

In this context, the nurse manager can also approach any problem with an individual caregiver who is always "doing it all," the one who provides total care all of the time. Education about the importance of active resident participation in ADL programming may need to be reviewed with even the best caregiver from time to time.

Transferring a resident out of a mid-stage Alzheimer's disease and related dementia program is a complex subject. Programming is designed specifically for the person at mid-stage, and without transfers, the programming becomes ineffective and eventually is set aside. When this occurs, "dementia-specific care" becomes a misnomer. The 31-day calendar of participation can support the social participation assessments done quarterly by the therapeutic recreation director. Keeping family members and staff advised of changes with these kinds of objective data can help them to gradually prepare for and reduce the trauma they feel when the time comes to determine that a resident is no longer benefitting from the social model of care offered in the program.

ADL CARE PLAN AND THE COMPUTER

The ADL Care Plan/Flow Sheet can easily be integrated into the computerized plan of care as follows.

Need/problem	Goals	Approaches
ADL deficit related to impaired cognition	Goal 1: verbal cuing and manual cuing for A.M. washing/disinfecting Goal 2: verbal cuing and manual cuing denture care	See ADL Care Plan

The ADL Care Plan/Flow Sheet can be removed from the licensed nursing assistant documentation books at the end of each month and placed with the computerized care plans in the care plan section of the medical record. ADL goals are printed on the quarterly report for the nurse's progress notes.

Special care issues related to ADLs can be incorporated into the care plan as separate problems, and the corresponding approaches can be entered. These will be printed on the LNA computer records. In this case, the ADL Care Plan/Flow Sheet will refer the caregiver to the computerized record with a note in the appropriate box, "See comp doc."

EFFECTING CHANGE IN A CLOSED UNIT

There should be something different about a special care program. One of the management issues is the sense of separateness that develops in these programs. Caregivers can be especially intimidated when an "outsider" enters to assess their work, and the outsider can be equally intimidated. The caregivers in these programs develop a strong sense of ownership and pride. When attempting to review the work being done in the program, it is important to establish a mood of mutual respect and to clarify early on the mutual goals of improving care while raising the consciousness of reimbursement issues. No one enjoys having his or her work analyzed by an "outsider." Not many enjoy the prospect of change. Improving a situation that seems to be working very well must be done with tact and sensitivity, avoiding any criticism of the fine work that has already been done.

In order to manage for high-quality outcomes, to monitor the cost of care under a magnifying glass, and to account for the minute details of care rendered, ownership must be given to and accepted by the clinical staff. This effort requires fine-tuned teamwork. It means that administrators and business managers must rely on the clinical staff in ways that are unfamiliar to them. It means that clinical staff must accept the challenge as part of their advocacy role and recognize it to be as important as any aspect of the care they provide.

How complicated is this effort for the staff? In and of itself, documenting is almost unnatural for nurturers. They would rather be "doing it" than "writing about it." In caring for residents with Alzheimer's disease and related disorders the staff have been taught to minimize disabilities and concentrate on the "can-dos," ignoring the "cannots." It is confusing for the nursing assistant who is now asked to document the maximum amount of assistance required throughout a 24-hour day. The staff naturally want to talk about, write about, and take credit for residents' successes, not residents' dependent needs. Staff must be given permission to do this. They need to know that this is not an admission of failure, but rather an acknowledgment of the characteristics of the disease itself.

I helped a team to organize and implement a special care program for the care of people with mid-stage dementia. The experience was exciting and successful, and the program was staffed by well-trained, dedicated caregivers. After 1 year, I returned to the program to complete a quality improvement project. Not surprisingly, a problem with transfers from the program and low case-mix scores had been identified. I knew the staff fairly well, having kept in touch with them through ongoing educational support. I had visited periodically to casually scan the environment, speak with the staff, and observe the programming. I kept such visits to a minimum to respect the philosophy of the low-traffic, low-stimulation closed program.

In this return visit, I felt as if I had entered an inner sanctum and I smiled with pleasure at my observations. Soft music was playing. Wanderers, going nowhere, greeted me with a smile. A rummager was safely rummaging through an antique desk. A program of reminiscence and another of exercise were keeping some residents busy. One lady in the kitchen was washing a dish repeatedly. She was smiling too.

My intention in returning was to compare the accuracy of documentation to actual care and to review our transfer criteria and procedures. Having previously announced that I would be visiting and asking for their help with a quality improvement project, I spoke with the staff and told them how pleased I was with what I saw. I tried to choose an inconspicuous corner to begin my review of the charts. There I observed the following:

> Mr. Morgan, 72 years old, sat at the dining room table staring out the window. After a few minutes, he succumbed to fatigue and rested his head on the table. Mr. Morgan was about 6 feet 2 inches tall and weighed 170 pounds. Programs were in progress all around him, but he ignored invitations to join in. It was not long before his caregiver, Sandy, approached him to take him to his bed.
>
> SANDY: John, do you want to go to bed?
> MR. MORGAN: [Raised his head from the table, but remained silent.]
> SANDY: Let me help you. [Attempted to assist him to his feet.]
> MR. MORGAN: [Smiled, but gave no verbal response.]
> SANDY: I'll be right back.
>
> Mr. Morgan put his head down again. Within minutes Sandy returned with a co-worker. Together they physically assisted Mr. Morgan to a standing position and walked him to his bed for a rest. I was pleased with their recognition of his need and of their approach. Then I opened his chart.

Mr. Morgan's record indicated that he was independent in ambulation and occasionally required verbal cuing for transfers. I felt I had to ask Sandy about the discrepancy between the documentation and her approach with Mr. Morgan.

GAIL: Sandy, are you Mr. Morgan's primary caregiver?
SANDY: Yes, he's *my* resident. [I got that message.]
GAIL: His chart indicates that he's pretty independent.
SANDY: That's right.
GAIL: [Cautiously] He just required a two-person assist.
SANDY: [Defensively] He gets tired in the afternoon.
GAIL: [Bravely] Every afternoon?
SANDY: [Patiently, but firmly] Yes. And I promised Mrs. Morgan that I would personally see that he got to bed for a nap when he got tired. Do you know Mrs. Morgan? [I got the message. *I* was the intruder.]
GAIL: Uh, no. But I can see that you know a great deal about Mr. and Mrs. Morgan's needs. Your approach was perfect. Could you help me review his chart and see what we need to do about the documentation?

Sandy agreed to help me and was obviously relieved that there was no need to defend her care. The incident was typical of what I discovered to be true about the gaps between actual care and documentation. The staff was recording what they had always recorded rather than the maximum assistance given during the shift.

Sandy and the other nursing assistants taught me many things. The system and the education we had provided were not adequate for case-mix needs. It was easy but far from accurate to place one's initials in a box to indicate that care was always provided in the same way. The wide variations in how the care was being rendered from shift to shift had already caused tension between the shifts. When the evening and night staff tried to document an increase in physical support, the day staff thought they were not doing enough cuing. I realized that the staff needed reeducation about sundowning and fatigue in Alzheimer's disease as well as a plan for intershift meetings.

A new documentation tool will not be successful overnight. It will take time to educate, to implement, to revise, and to monitor—not once or twice, but continually. Do not minimize the effect of staff turnover rates in nursing facilities. Many good programs are lost through attrition when new policies and procedures are not integrated into orientation and basic education programs.

Adding new documentation tools may not be easy, but it is definitely worthwhile. Every effort should be made to nurture and tend with this practice.

REHABILITATION, CASE-MIX, AND THE RESIDENT WITH ALZHEIMER'S DISEASE

Individuals diagnosed with Alzheimer's disease and related disorders can be difficult to assess for secondary conditions that can affect their function. At the same time, advancing age puts many individuals at high risk for multiple health problems.

It is not unusual to see swallowing problems, falls (with or without fractures), or declines in ambulation skills as early symptoms of a secondary condition. It is not only acceptable to access the rehabilitation team, it is mandated for by federal law. Many providers have been rejected for Part B Medicare because the therapists have used dementia as a primary diagnosis. More success has been attained when billing with the International Classification of Diseases-9 (ICD-9) code that best describes the primary reason for the specific therapy. Realistic expectations and duration of therapy must be set with acknowledgment of the individual's cognitive losses.

During rehabilitation, the MDS+ may capture the Low Intensity Rehab category and improve the case-mix score. The resident and family benefit with improved function or additional safety measures taken. If there is no improvement, they at least have the satisfaction of knowing that every reasonable effort was made on their behalf. The facility has documentation so that surveyors can see that the decline in function was related to the disease process and not to neglect.

CHALLENGING BEHAVIORS

Occasionally, a person with early-stage Alzheimer's disease is admitted to a nursing facility. This can happen when there is a lack of family caregivers, a shortage of beds in residential care, and commonly when the disease attacks the person's awareness of his or her safety in the early stage. If, after a period of adjustment, the resident falls into a 1.0 case-mix score, the staff should be alerted. It is unlikely that the resident is cured of his or her behaviors. It is more likely that the staff have planned for and accepted the behaviors. With proper documentation of this "light care" resident's behaviors, the Vermont case-mix classification system would move him or her to a score of 1.21. The behavior flow sheet used should be reviewed to be certain that each behavior pertinent to the state's case-mix system and the MDS+ is included for easy documentation.

Well-trained caregivers have a way of becoming blind to inappropriate behaviors. After all, they are taught to minimize the behaviors. They are taught techniques to avoid catastrophic reactions, and they function in an environment designed for safety. It is fairly common to hear staff responses that defend behavior, such as, "not unusual for her . . . she always does that . . . no one got hurt." It can be helpful to ask the staff to picture the behavior in a theater or in church and to assess again how appropriate it is. This frequently evokes a smile and a nod of agreement.

Staff need education in the behaviors as defined very specifically in the MDS+ document. These are the behaviors that will be factored into the case-mix score. Wandering, described in the MDS+ as moving "with no rational purpose; seemingly oblivious to needs or safety," seems to be particularly difficult for the staff to assess. Going to an alarmed door, even when intercepted and redirected, is wandering. Pacing is wandering. It is not unusual for a wanderer to require limited physical assistance for purposeful ambulation, for example, to meals or to toilet. Wandering can be ignored in the safe environment of a closed program. It can also be mistaken for independent, purposeful transfer activity and can reduce the case-mix score.

Verbal and physical abuse can also be overlooked. The staff learn to accept aggressive behaviors from some residents, and by applying principles of nonconfrontational care, they manage to avert catastrophic reactions. In the absence of disaster and/or injury, the behavior frequently goes undocumented.

Many caregivers cannot define, much less document, delusional thinking. Yet it is a very common symptom among residents. Caring for someone who is displaying delusional behavior can require a great deal of skill and time by the caregiver.

If maximum case-mix scores are missed because of poor documentation in the area of behaviors, much can be placed at risk. The safety features of the program that prevent wandering off the grounds, the concentrated individualized programs, and well-educated staff (available and flexible to deal with the unexpected) all cost money.

CONCLUSIONS

What the future holds for reimbursement in nursing facilities is a bit of an enigma. Some observers believe that case-mix is here to stay in one form or another. Other observers believe that it will be replaced as managed care groups buy Medicaid and Medicare contracts. Still others believe capitated payment will drive the health care system in ways yet to be imagined.

Whichever way it goes, it is certain that accountability will be a major factor. Providing the around-the-clock needs of the resident with Alzheimer's disease and related disorders will continue to be a challenge, and detailed documentation may be the only defense of staffing needs and other costs of special care programs.

REFERENCES

Minimum data set plus for nursing home resident assessment and care plan screening (MDS+).

Romano, M. (1994, May). All mixed up. *Contemporary Long-Term Care*, pp. 40–42.

Roy, J. (1995). *Hypothetical case-mix analysis.* Bennington, VT: Weston Hadden Convalescent Center.

Vermont Agency of Human Services. (1991). *Case-mix classification workbook.* Montpelier, VT: Author.

10

Research Update in Alzheimer's Disease

Jonathan B. Hoyne, B.A., Dani Fallin, B.S.,
and Michael J. Mullan, M.D., Ph.D., M.R.C.Psych.

Alzheimer's disease is a common dementing mental disorder, characterized clinically by a continual loss of cognitive functioning and pathologically by cortical deposition of amyloid (waxy translucent, hard proteins that are deposited in organs and tissues under abnormal conditions) plaques and the development of neurofibrillary tangles as well as neuron death. This disease is often subdivided based on age at disease onset. The line between early and late onset is arbitrarily set at 65 years, with early-onset familial cases being caused by genetic mutations and late-onset cases being caused by many factors.

Whatever the cause, time from onset to death is highly variable among individuals but averages about 7 years (Gustafson, 1992). The relentless progression and extended course of Alzheimer's disease inflict both a psychological and economic toll on the spouse or primary caregiver, generally requiring full-time medical treatment in the final stages. In addition, incidence of the disease rises to about 25%–45% at 85 years of age (Breteler, Claus, van Duijn, Launer, & Hofman, 1992). The prevalence of an extended and thoroughly debilitating disease such as Alzheimer's disease in a population that is growing because of longer life expectancy will exact a high price from American society. In light of this fact, extensive research on a variety of fronts attracts significant amounts of government funding.

Since the mid-1970s, research has steadily advanced our understanding of Alzheimer's disease (Fratiglioni, 1993). However, there is no single theory as to the cause of the majority of cases. Drug treatments are still unable to halt or reliably slow the disease process.

CLINICAL DESCRIPTION

The first symptoms of Alzheimer's disease are usually manifested by an inability to recall recently learned material as well as by an inability to learn new skills. This early stage may not be noticed until revealed by a stressor, such as declining job performance or a major change in lifestyle (Mullan & Brown, 1994). Often, the exact time of onset of the disease is difficult to pinpoint. Initially some affected individuals retain insight into their disability, which may produce secondary depression that usually subsides as cognitive decline continues and insight is lost. This phase of the disease may last as long as 2–3 years, during which time the patient and family members adjust to these new circumstances. Individuals display progressive intellectual decline in tests of cognitive functioning (Mullan & Brown, 1994) in the first few years, reflecting an underlying cumulative and progressive neuropathological process.

As the disease progresses global functioning is increasingly impaired. In the second stage of the disease apraxia (inability to make purposeful movements that is not caused by paralysis), aphasia (deficit or loss of speech), agnosia (loss of the ability to recognize the meaning of stimuli), and loss of executive abilities (e.g., organizing, planning, making judgments) are common. The person increasingly loses the capacity for complex behavior, including many activities of daily living (ADLs) (American Psychiatric Association, 1994). Individuals may engage in wandering and confrontational behaviors. Delusions may be common, particularly those involving possessions that the person believes are stolen, but are actually misplaced (Mullan, 1993). Changes in personality may be reflected in a broad spectrum of behaviors. Disinhibition may occur with inappropriate social and sexual interactions. Apathy, self-neglect, and decreased activity may also be evident. Some individuals may display motor impairment with the onset of parkinsonian features (e.g., gait disturbance, tremor), myoclonus (muscular rigidity), and seizures (Risse et al., 1990).

In the final stage people with Alzheimer's disease require total care as they lose coordinated motor control and sphincter control, which causes bladder and bowel incontinence. They become susceptible to injury and usually die from complications associated with immobility (e.g., bronchopneumonia, septicemia).

COST TO SOCIETY

As a result of the debilitating nature of Alzheimer's disease, affected individuals receive extensive care, sometimes from health care personnel, more frequently from family members, and often from both. A variety of contributing factors must be considered (e.g., prevalence rates, population size, care setting, length of postonset survival) when calculating the total financial cost of this care.

One study used midrange values for each contributing factor and determined annual Alzheimer's disease costs for 1991 in excess of $47,000 per person and $67 billion for Americans overall (Ernst & Hay, 1994). These estimates include loss of income by caregivers as well as other indirect costs. Assuming that these numbers are even reasonably accurate, the savings from a small advance in Alzheimer's disease research could be substantial.

DIAGNOSTIC CRITERIA

Making the diagnosis of Alzheimer's disease is problematic as a result of the variety of diagnoses that present in a similar manner. The diagnosis is based on either the criteria outlined in the *Diagnostic and Statistical Manual of Mental Disorders* (4th ed.) (American Psychiatric Association, 1994) or the criteria set forth by the U.S. National Institute for Neurological and Communicative Disorders and Stroke (NINCDS) and the Alzheimer's Disease and Related Disorders Association (ADRDA) (McKahnn, Drachman, Folstein, Datzman, Price, & Stadlan, 1984).

A diagnosis of Alzheimer's disease is made only when all other possible diagnoses are excluded. Competing diagnoses include vascular dementia, dementia as a result of head trauma, substance-induced persisting dementia, and dementia as a result of diseases (e.g., Parkinson disease, Huntington disease, AIDS, Pick disease, Creutzfeldt-Jakob disease). The person's history and a variety of clinical tests (e.g., blood tests, electrocardiogram, chest x ray, and electroencephalogram) are also utilized. With a positive diagnosis of Alzheimer's disease, the diagnosing physician may further delineate the disease into one of several subcategories.

The criteria in DSM-IV (1994) outline Dementia of the Alzheimer's Type subcategories based on the age of onset. An additional set of subcategories indicate the predominant feature of the current clinical presentation—Dementia of the Alzheimer's Type with delirium, with delusions, with depressed mood, or uncomplicated.

NINCDS criteria outline subcategories based on the certainty of diagnosis. The three categories are possible, probable, and definite Alzheimer's disease. A diagnosis of possible Alzheimer's disease is assigned when dementia is established by the appropriate neuropsychiatric scale (e.g., Mini-Mental State Examination, Blessed Dementia Scale) with age of onset from 40 to 90 (usually after age 65), no disturbance of consciousness, deficits in at least two areas of cognition, and progressive deterioration of memory. Possible dementia can also be diagnosed in the presence of a second dementing process (e.g., small strokes) that is not sufficiently severe to be the sole cause of the observed cognitive deficits. Also present are progressive deterioration in language, motor skills, or perception; a family history of Alzheimer's disease (particularly if it has been confirmed postmortem); impairment in ability to perform ADLs; normal lumbar puncture and electroencephalogram results; and serial computed tomography scans showing progressive cerebral atrophy.

Both DSM-IV (1994) and NINCDS require the exclusion of all other possible causes of the observed cognitive deficits. A diagnosis of definite Alzheimer's disease is made only when there is postmortem pathological confirmation of the disease, and the person was assigned a diagnosis of probable Alzheimer's disease in life. However, many clinicians can accurately (>85%) diagnose Alzheimer's disease while the person is alive.

Upon microscopic examination, a necessary, although not sufficient, pathologic feature of the disease is the deposit of amyloid in dense extracellular plaques. However, amyloid plaques have been identified in cognitively normal older individuals, suggesting that whereas their formation is a central feature of Alzheimer's disease, they may not be causative (Delaere et al., 1990).

Neurofibrillary tangles, another classic neuropathologic feature, are abnormal neural bodies that contain paired spiral filaments (Alzheimer, 1906, 1907a, 1907b). Additional pathologic characteristics include neuronal loss and glial cell death (Katzman & Thal, 1989).

EPIDEMIOLOGY

Prevalence/Incidence

Prevalence (the number of individuals in a given population who have the disease during a specified time period) is dependent upon incidence (the number of new cases per time period) and the duration of the disease after onset. Prevalence estimates help to assess the relative impact a disease will have on a community rather than to determine the etiology of the disease. Estimation of incidence rates, however, can be stratified by age, gender, or any other factor that may suggest possible origins of the disease.

Prevalence estimates of Alzheimer's disease vary greatly, yet all studies show that prevalence increases with age. In a collaborative study comparing age-dependent prevalence rates from six European studies Rocca et al. (1991) combined community-based studies with equivalent diagnostic criteria. The pooled prevalence estimate was then broken into age groups as follows: 0.4% for women and 0.3% for men age 60–69, 3.6%

for women and 2.5% for men age 70–79, 11.2% for women and 10% for men age 80–89, and 24.7% for women and 40.9% for men age 90 and over. (*Note:* The 90 and over age group estimate was based on only one study.) The differences seen between this analysis and American studies may be due in part to the use of different methodologies (Jorm, Dorten, & Henderson, 1987; Rocca, Amaducci, & Schoenberg, 1986).

The incidence of Alzheimer's disease was estimated in a study (Kokmen, Chandra, & Schoenberg, 1988; Schoenberg, Kokmen, & Okazaki, 1987) as 66 per 100,000 people per year in the 60–65 age group. This increased to 409 in the 70–79 age group and to 1,480 for all individuals ≥80 years old. Although much higher incidence rates were seen in Sweden and France—115 per 100,000 people in the 60–69 age group, 600 in the 70–79 age group, and 2,230 in the 80 and above age group (Dartigues et al., 1992; Rorsman, Hagnell, & Lanke, 1986)—the findings of most other studies place rates between these two extremes. Again, as with prevalence, incidence increases with age.

The prevalence of Alzheimer's disease and related disorders was consistent across countries, with the exceptions of China and Japan, which showed a larger group with vascular dementia and a smaller group with Alzheimer's disease. Smaller Alzheimer's disease prevalence rates were revealed for Japan than for any of the European or American data sets. These data were consistent with previous data on prevalence rates in Japan as well as China (Jorm, 1991).

An investigation into the nature of this discrepancy used American-trained psychiatrists diagnosing individuals with dementia in Shanghai (Zhang, Datzman, & Salmon, 1990). The relative prevalence rates of vascular dementia and Alzheimer's disease closely correlated with the American studies, suggesting that the difference in prevalence observed between the Chinese population and the American and European populations is the result of differential application of diagnostic criteria.

Risk Factors

The search for biological risk factors has included exposure to aluminum and lead, age, gender, medical history (mainly head injury, psychiatric disorders, thyroid problems, and anesthesia), family history of dementia, family history of Down syndrome or Parkinson disease, tobacco and alcohol use, occupational exposures to solvents, and others. The research into each of these factors has been problematic, resulting in conflicting and inconclusive epidemiological findings. The most notable of these studies are discussed in the following sections.

European Community Concerned Action Epidemiology and Prevention of Dementia (EURODEM) Studies Van Duijn, Stijnen, and Hofman (1994) conducted an analysis of 11 large case-control studies (1960–1988) reported from six different countries in which they evaluated risk factors from six major categories—family history of dementia, parental age at birth, medical history, psychiatric history, alcohol and tobacco use, and occupational exposure to solvents and lead. Among these factors, only four were found to be key risks significantly associated with Alzheimer's disease: positive family history of Alzheimer's disease, a history of head injury, a history of depression, and the presence of Down syndrome in a family. Of these key factors, positive family history carried the greatest risk for Alzheimer's disease.

Most of the EURODEM studies showed a positive, although not conclusive, association between head trauma and Alzheimer's disease (Amaducci et al., 1986; Chandra, Kokmen, Schoenberg, & Beard, 1989; van Duijn, Stijnen, & Hofman, 1994). The association reached significance only when the data from these studies were combined (Chandra et al., 1989; van Duijn et al., 1994). In the pooled estimate, the incidence of Alzheimer's disease among individuals with head injury was 47% higher than in the control population. This association is supported by the observation of neurofibrillary tangles in dementia pugilistica, a dementing illness in boxers that results from the cumulative effects of repeated minor head traumas.

Five of six EURODEM studies showed a positive risk for individuals with a history of depression, both immediately preceding Alzheimer's disease onset and much earlier in life. In the grouped analysis of EURODEM studies individuals with an immediate family member with Down syndrome were 2.7 times more likely than individuals without to develop Alzheimer's disease. This effect was strongest in people who also had a family history of dementia.

Gender and Estrogen Several studies have reported a higher prevalence of Alzheimer's disease in women than in men (Kokmen, Beard, & Offord, 1989; Rocca et al., 1990; O'Connor, Pollitt, & Hyde, 1989). Studies investigating survival time from disease onset have reported an extended duration of the disease in women (Diesfeldt, van Houten, & Moerkens, 1986; Heyman, Wilkinson, & Hurwitz, 1987). This increased prevalence in women may be a result of their extended survival rather than a true gender difference.

The association of survival time led to the study of estrogen in the disease process. Paganini-Hill and Henderson (1994) reported that postmenopausal women on estrogen replacement therapy had a decreased incidence of the disease as compared to the control group. In addition, estrogen users with Alzheimer's disease showed significantly less cognitive decline than did females with Alzheimer's disease who were not taking estrogen (Henderson, Paganini-Hill, Emanuel, Dunn, & Buckwalter, 1994). These studies may support a role for estrogen as a neural growth factor (Honjo, Tamura, Matsumoto, Dawata, & Ogino, 1992). The mechanism of estrogen's effect on Alzheimer's disease is not understood. Many research projects, including projects supported by the National Institute on Aging, are aimed at investigating the relationship between estrogen and Alzheimer's disease (Mulnard et al., 1995).

Anesthesia Frequent anecdotal reports of rapid decline in individuals with Alzheimer's disease following exposure to anesthesia have raised the question of an association between the two. This notion is supported by the observation that anesthesia can have a prolonged effect on postoperative mental functioning in normal patients (Jones, 1989). However, the EURODEM reanalysis of studies assessing anesthesia as a risk factor for Alzheimer's disease failed to reveal a significant association (Amaducci et al., 1986; Broe et al., 1990; Graves et al., 1990a; van Duijn et al., 1994). In addition, a recent study by Bohnen, Warner, Kokmen, Beard, and Kurland (1994) showed no effect of cumulative exposure to anesthesia on the incidence of Alzheimer's disease.

Aluminum Several studies investigated aluminum exposure because aluminum silicates are found in individuals with Alzheimer's disease in amyloid plaques as well as in neurons containing neurofibrillary tangles. Correlations were reported between aluminum in drinking water and Alzheimer's disease (Breteler et al., 1992; Martyn & Barker, 1989). However, drinking water contributes only a small amount of aluminum to an individual's total intake, and studies evaluating the effect of aluminum intake from a variety of sources produced conflicting data. Some studies reported no association even in subjects who had been exposed to high doses (Foncin, 1987). Similarly, studies of individuals who took antacids containing aluminum failed to show a correlation with Alzheimer's disease in this group (Graves et al., 1990b). Furthermore, the majority of studies that did report an aluminum-associated risk have been criticized (Breteler et al., 1992) for employing poor diagnostic criteria of affected individuals that were unrepresentative of the typical clinical diagnostic criteria (Martyn & Barker, 1989). As a result of these problems, no firm conclusion can yet be reached, and further study is required to fully explain any possible connection that exists.

Age Overall, the factor most associated with Alzheimer's disease is advancing age. Onset of the disease is age dependent; very few cases below age 35 have been reported. Furthermore, the risk of the disease for any individual increases even into the 9th and 10th decades (O'Connor, Pollitt, & Hyde, 1989).

Summary

It seems almost certain that environmental factors play a role in Alzheimer's disease. However, these factors must be ubiquitous, as aging populations from diverse geographic areas have approximately the same age-related prevalence rates. Many research groups have concentrated on identifying genetic factors that are specifically predisposing.

GENETIC STUDIES

Early-Onset Alzheimer's Disease

Early-onset familial Alzheimer's disease shows a pattern of inheritance that is consistent with transmission of a dominant gene. This fact has led to the investigation of the role of genetics in early-onset disease etiology.

Clinical Manifestations Familial early-onset studies have thus far revealed two causative loci as well as the possibility of a third (Lannfelt et al., 1993; Schellenberg et al., 1988, 1992). Whereas these cases have genetically distinct etiologies, they result in remarkably similar clinical presentation and pathology (Mullan et al., 1993; Mullan et al., 1994). The most striking clinical difference between etiologies occurs in the age at disease onset. Families with chromosome 14 abnormalities display an age of onset in the 40s, whereas chromosome 21 families (with β-APP mutations) develop the disease slightly later, in their mid-50s (Mullan et al., 1993). A third early-onset locus has been identified on chromosome 1, which accounts for familial disease with ages of onset ranging from the 50s to the 70s (Levy-Lahad et al., 1995).

All forms of early-onset Alzheimer's disease are otherwise typical clinically, presenting with an insidious progression. Short-term memory loss is the earliest sign. Subsequently, global loss of cognitive functioning progresses steadily. Individuals in some families with chromosome 21–linked onset progress with a slight increase in early dyspraxia (impairment in ability to perform coordinated movements), dysphasia (inability to link words together in their proper order), and dyscalculia (impaired ability to perform simple mathematical problems). In one of these families, headaches were a common preclinical symptom (Mullan et al., 1994).

Both subsets of early-onset Alzheimer's disease are more striking in their clinical similarity to typical Alzheimer's disease than in any gross differences. The presence of a distinct age of onset difference in these families provides a convenient clinical screening tool for preliminary classification of individuals with likely chromosome 21– or chromosome 14–linked families.

Chromosome 21 The observation that individuals with Down syndrome (trisomy 21) who survive into their 40s always develop Alzheimer's disease pathology led to the investigation of the role of chromosome 21 in Alzheimer's disease development (Glenner & Wong, 1984). β-Amyloid precursor protein gene (β-APP), a protein that can lead to the formation of the amyloid plaques found in Alzheimer's disease, was subsequently localized on chromosome 21 (Goldgaber, Lerman, McBride, Saffiotti, &

Gajdusek, 1987; Tanzi, Gusella, Watkins, Bruns, & St. George-Hyslop, 1987). Because of the multiple genetic causes of familial Alzheimer's disease, the β-APP gene was initially overlooked as a cause of Alzheimer's disease. The classification of Alzheimer's disease cases based on disease onset (St. George-Hyslop, Haines, & Farrer, 1990) allowed researchers to identify a subset of cases in which mutations at β-APP cause the disease (Chartier-Harlin et al., 1991; Goate, Rossor, Roques, Hardy, & Mullan, 1991; Mullan, Houlden, Windelspecht, Fidani, & Lombardi, 1992; Murrell, Farlow, Ghetti, & Benson, 1991). This finding represents the first known cause of Alzheimer's disease.

Transfection and Transgenic Studies Although familial early-onset cases comprise only about 20% of all familial Alzheimer's disease, these mutations represent a powerful tool for further molecular studies into the disease. By incorporating the mutations in transfection (incorporating the gene into living cell cultures) and transgenic (incorporating the gene into germ line cells, which results in an animal's carrying one or more copies of the gene) studies, intensive investigation of the molecular pathology of Alzheimer's disease is now possible. Additionally, the use of these mutations in animals is likely to expedite the development of potent pharmacological treatments.

Summary Work on genetic errors that lead to early-onset Alzheimer's disease has provided strong clues to the mechanism of the disease process. The inclusion of some other trigger associated with age should not be overlooked when modeling the disease process. The challenge is to determine the physiologic function of the proteins coded for these known Alzheimer's disease genes.

Late-Onset Alzheimer's Disease

Although 80% of cases have onset after age 65, no causative locus for late-onset Alzheimer's disease has been found. The occurrence of families who have many family members with late-onset Alzheimer's disease has interested researchers in investigating the genetic cause. However, it is unlikely that one gene causes the majority of late-onset cases. A better model includes the possibility of multigene transmission, genetic heterogeneity, and environmental factors in late-onset Alzheimer's disease. Some studies have supported this theory.

Association of the apolipoprotein CII gene in sporadic, late-onset Alzheimer's disease first implicated chromosome 19 (Schellenberg et al., 1987). A locus in this area has been identified as the gene coding apolipoprotein E. Apolipoprotein E is the protein component of one of the plasma lipoproteins whose main physiologic role is the metabolism and transport of lipids. Strittmatter et al. (1993) found an increase in the frequency of the E4 allele (form) of the apolipoprotein E gene from 16% in controls to 50% in individuals with late-onset Alzheimer's disease. This observation of increased frequency of the E4 allele has since been replicated by many groups (Bennett et al., 1995; Noguchi, Murakaami, & Yamada, 1993; Porier, Davignon, Bouthillier, Kogan, Bertrand, & Gauthier, 1993; Rebeck, Reiter, Strickland, & Hyman, 1993).

Relationship of Apolipoprotein E to Alzheimer's Disease By examining the relationship between the apolipoprotein E genotype and the occurrence of the disease, Bennett et al. (1995) showed that apolipoprotein E was a poor predictor of disease status within families with multiply affected late-onset Alzheimer's disease, but the same trend of an excess percentage of the E4 allele in all affected individuals was still valid. Combining these data, Bennett and co-workers (1995) proposed a model that explains the distortion of apolipoprotein E alleles in late-onset Alzheimer's disease. By exerting an influence on rate of disease progression, the E4 allele could allow individuals to cross the clinical threshold earlier than they would otherwise (as seen by the dose effect). This appears to have been validated in 1995 by a Finnish study that failed to find an association between the E4 allele and late-onset Alzheimer's disease in affected centenarians (Sobel et al., 1995). Furthermore, this model predicts that in a sample of cognitively normal older individuals, the frequency of occurrence of the E4 allele will decrease as a function of age. Rebeck, Perls, West, Sodhi, Lipsitz, and Hyman (1994) have observed this expected decrease in the E4 allele.

The evidence examined earlier, the existence of several cognitively normal homozygous individuals identified by the authors' group, and the existence of a 100-year-old person with two copies of the E4 allele (Sobel et al., 1995) suggest that apolipoprotein E is not sufficient to cause late-onset Alzheimer's disease. Rather, variants may affect the rate of the disease process once it has begun. The physiologic mechanism by which apolipoprotein E accomplishes this is an area of intense scientific inquiry. An example is seen in early-onset families. St. George-Hyslop et al. (1994) demonstrated that the age of onset of members of β-APP families is modified by their apolipoprotein E genotype. These families had presented with an age of onset in the mid 50s. Within these families, individuals with a copy of the E4 allele presented with an earlier age of onset, in the late 40s. Investigation into a similar effect in families with onset linked to chromosome 14 failed to observe a similar effect (Van Broeckhoven et al., 1994), which is consistent with the previous observation of little variability in disease onset for these families (Mullan et al., 1993). It appears that apolipoprotein E can influence the age of onset in otherwise predisposed individuals.

Proposed Physiologic Mechanisms of Apolipoprotein E A clue to the physiologic mechanism of apolipoprotein E may lie in the localization of apolipoprotein E with amyloid plaques. Other possible physiologic mechanisms have also been advanced. Through its role as a lipid transport molecule and as the primary lipoprotein expressed in the brain, apolipoprotein E has been implicated in neural regeneration by redistributing lipids both during neurite extension and to specialized cells during remyelination. In vitro studies of apolipoprotein E physiology have shown that cholesterol-associated apolipoprotein E stimulates neural branching (Handelman, Boyles, Weisgraber, Mahley, & Pitas, 1992). Physiologic roles are possible, as indicated above, by which E4 might enhance the Alzheimer's disease process.

TREATMENT STRATEGIES

Our most complete understanding of Alzheimer's disease will be a description of the disease process at the molecular level. Incomplete understanding of the disease is likely to give rise to therapies with only partial efficacy. For example, the model of cholinergic loss explains only a part of the biochemical abnormalities in Alzheimer's disease.

Anticholinesterase Therapies

In the development of drug therapies for Alzheimer's disease, attention has been focused on the cholinergic hypothesis first proposed by Bartus and colleagues in 1982 (Bartus, Dean, Beer, & Lippa, 1982). They suggested that the forebrain acetylcholine system is the basis for a number of cognitive processes (mainly memory and learning), and that a decline in the functional capability of this system correlates with a clinical decline in memory and learning abilities. Coyle, Price, & DeLong (1983) adapted this theory to Alzheimer's disease specifically for three reasons: 1) the notable loss of acetylcholine and the enzyme that produces it in individuals with Alzheimer's disease, 2) the correlation between biochemical measures of the acetylcholine systems and clinical decline in people with Alzheimer's disease, and 3) the loss or atrophy of basal forebrain neurons in individuals with Alzheimer's disease (Dunnett & Fibiger, 1993).

From the findings delineated in the previous paragraph two possible treatment strategies involving the cholinergic system emerged. First, choline precursor drugs were suggested, specifically lecithin, that would increase the amount of extracellular choline, a precursor to acetylcholine (Giacobini, 1993). This approach was used in some clinical trials and was relatively unsuccessful (Whitehouse, 1993). A second and much more promising approach used inhibitors of the enzyme acetylcholinesterase, which breaks down acetylcholine and thus increases the overall amount of acetylcholine. Early studies included physostigmine, which showed promise but had a short half-life, making it difficult to maintain therapeutic serum levels over time. This trial was followed by trials with many other acetylcholinesterase inhibitors, including pyridostigmine, heptylphysostigmine, galanthamine, epigalanthamine, metrifonate, huperzine A, velnacrine, tacrine, SDZ ENA 713, SM-10888, NIK-247, and MDL

73745, most of which are still in clinical trials. Only tacrine tetrahydroaminoacridine, brand name Cognex) has been approved by the U.S. Food and Drug Administration.

Tacrine has been the most effective inhibitor of acetylcholinesterase, showing an improvement in cognitive functioning and prolonged increase in acetylcholine in individuals with Alzheimer's disease as compared to a placebo (Chatellier & Lacomblez, 1990; Eagger, Levy, & Sahakian, 1991; Gauthier, Bouchard, Lamontagne, Bailey, & Bergman, 1990; Molloy, Guyatt, Wilson, Duke, Rees, & Singer, 1991). In three of five clinical trials conducted between 1986 and 1991, patients taking tacrine showed significant improvement in cognitive, functional, and behavioral scales. The other two trials showed no improvement. Comparison across these studies is difficult as a result of the variety of measurement tools used.

A large, multicenter trial showed tacrine to significantly improve cognitive function in individuals with Alzheimer's disease (Davis et al., 1992). The trial was a 12-week, double-blind, placebo-controlled study of 468 patients with Alzheimer's disease. From this group, 159 subjects were discontinued as a result of adverse effects (see following paragraph). Of the 273 patients who completed this study, 130 showed cognitive improvement.

Tacrine may cause severe elevation of liver enzymes as well as other side effects, including nausea and/or vomiting, diarrhea, abdominal pain, dyspepsia, and rash (Beerman, 1993; Wolf-Klein, 1993). These effects are highly dependent on the age and concomitant disease status of the individual. The consensus is that people in the early to middle stages of Alzheimer's disease are expected to benefit from tacrine, and the most efficacious dosage appears to be 40 mg/day for 6 weeks and then 80 mg/day for the following 6 weeks. Maintenance dosage and long-term effects of tacrine therapy are presently unknown.

The drug SDZ ENA 713, a nicotinic derivative that blocks acetylcholinesterase both in vitro and in vivo, is being studied because of its selectivity for the brain, its prolonged activity, and its apparent tolerability (Enz, Amstutz, Boddeke, Gmelin, & Malanowski, 1993). Not until large clinical trials of this drug are completed will the efficacy of this new drug be determined and compared to the now-standard tacrine therapy.

Nerve Growth Factor

The possibility of nerve growth factor as a palliative therapy in Alzheimer's disease is based on the observation that supplying exogenous nerve growth factor in animal models with degeneration of basal forebrain cholinergic neurons has an ameliorating effect on tests of cognitive functioning (Fischer, Wictorin, Bjorklund, Williams, Varon, & Gage, 1987). These neurons are selectively affected in Alzheimer's disease, and therefore replication of this effect in humans may slow cognitive decline in the disease.

One complication of using nerve growth factor as a therapy is the difficulty of delivery to the brain. Many of these molecules are either too large or have electrical properties that prevent them from penetrating the blood–brain barrier. Delivery strategies fall into a number of categories, two of which are of particular importance: direct introduction of nerve growth factor into the brain through a surgically implanted pump and carrier-mediated transport, coupling nerve growth factor with a molecule capable of penetrating the blood–brain barrier. Alternatively, nerve growth factor–inducing compounds (many of which readily pass the blood–brain barrier) are being investigated.

More trials are needed to assess the efficacy of nerve growth factor treatment. The manipulation of nerve growth factors in vivo is likely to be difficult. No simple solution exists to a complex etiologic problem such as Alzheimer's disease.

Inflammatory Mechanisms

A variety of immunoreactive proteins is found during postmortem analysis of the brain in Alzheimer's disease, which are absent or expressed at very low levels in the normal brain (McGeer, Akiyama, Itagaki, & McGeer, 1989). Among these proteins are α_1-antichymotrypsin and α_2-macroglobulin, which are associated with the inflammatory acute-phase response and are found in amyloid plaques. This finding has spurred interest in inflammatory mechanisms that may be active in Alzheimer's disease. The observation that the disease is relatively rare in people affected with rheumatoid arthritis helped advance the hypothesis that treatment with antiinflammatory drugs may be a prophylactic treatment for Alzheimer's disease and thus has led to further studies of treatment effects with antiinflammatory drugs (Breitner et al., 1994; Li, Shen, Chen, Zhau, & Silverman, 1992).

In a study by Rich, Rasmusson, Folstein, Carson, Kawas, & Brandt (1995), 32 of 210 patients with Alzheimer's disease were interviewed retrospectively and found to be taking nonsteroidal antiinflammatory drugs. All patients were then given a comprehensive physical and mental status examination, which were repeated at 1-year follow-up. Scores on some of these scales (Mini-Mental State Examination, Category Fluency Test, Boston Naming Test, Gollin Incomplete Figures Test) were significantly lower for those in the nonsteroidal antiinflammatory drug group. At the 1-year follow-up, patients in the nonsteroidal antiinflammatory drug group showed less decline on Mini-Mental State Examination scores than did those in the control group, despite the fact that overall those with high Mini-Mental State Examination scores showed the greatest decline. Many other cognitive tests were administered that did not reveal statistically significant differences between nonsteroidal antiinflammatory drugs and control subjects. However, all variables did show reliable differences in mean scores between groups in the direction predicted. Another study utilizing the co-twin control method sampled 50 pairs of twins discordant for Alzheimer's disease (either one twin was unaffected or the age of onset differed by at least 3 years). An inverse relationship was found between status with regard to Alzheimer's disease and previous treatment with nonsteroidal antiinflammatory drugs (Breitner et al., 1994).

The single prospective clinical trial in this area compared cognitive performance of subjects taking the nonsteroidal antiinflammatory drug indomethacin with a control group taking a placebo (Rogers et al., 1993). At 6-month follow-up, there was a statistically significant difference between the groups—a 1.3% increase on Mini-Mental State Examination scores in the indomethacin group, whereas the placebo group decreased 8.3%.

PRECLINICAL TESTING

Much research has focused on the development of tests to definitively identify Alzheimer's disease, particularly when signs of cognitive decline are the least obvious. Several different areas have been explored.

Eye Testing

One of the most promising testing procedures was reported by Scinto and colleagues in 1994 utilizing a simple screening procedure that correctly identified 18 out of 19 individuals suspected to have Alzheimer's disease (Scinto et al., 1994). In a control sample of older individuals from community living facilities only 2 of 32 exhibited a significant reaction consistent with proposed prevalence rates of Alzheimer's disease in this population. Furthermore, the response of individuals diagnosed with non-Alzheimer's disease dementia was similar to that of normal controls. The screening procedure requires the administration of a drop of tropicamide into the person's eye. In people affected with Alzheimer's disease, administration of this drug induces dilation of the pupil significantly greater than that induced in controls. Maximum sensitivity and specificity are attained by taking readings 29 minutes postadministration.

Further testing of this procedure with larger epidemiological samples is of primary importance to provide a convenient, rapid, and relatively inexpensive screening measure capable of delineating Alzheimer's and non-Alzheimer's dementias and of identifying cognitively normal people.

Genetic Testing

In a few cases genetic testing provides definitive preclinical (even prenatal) diagnosis of Alzheimer's disease. However, because the number of cases of Alzheimer's disease that are completely determined by aberrant genes is so small, genetic information for the average individual with Alzheimer's disease is less useful. The few families with known genetic mutations for early onset to whom this genetic testing does apply can now easily be screened, and affected individuals can be identified many years prior to age of onset. When releasing this genetic information, important ethical issues arise that require professional genetic counseling. Theoretically, this knowledge could be helpful if a prophylactic treatment is found that could delay onset. For now, its usefulness lies in social and economic preparations for people who are genetically at risk.

Genetic testing for the late-onset form of the disease is more problematic. Most cases of late-onset disease are not familial, and those that are familial do not transmit known mutations. To date, apolipoprotein E is the only genetic locus useful for late-onset disease prediction, although other loci have been reported to enhance its association (Kamboh, Sanghera, Ferrell, & DeKosky, 1995; Okuizumi et al., 1995). With the poor correlation between apolipoprotein E variants and Alzheimer's disease affection status, estimation of an individual's relative risk for the disease, given his or her apolipoprotein E genotype, can be based only on allele frequencies from large populations. In any specific case there could be considerable differences between this predicted risk and the actual risk for that individual.

From a technical perspective, apolipoprotein E testing is likely to be used in the following way. Based on genotype, an individual's risk for developing Alzheimer's disease in a specific age range will be calculated. Gender and ethnic origin may influence these results. From this calculation, individuals will be told their chances of developing the disease in a particular time frame. How might this knowledge be useful? One way is that differences in apolipoprotein E genotype may be associated with better outcome in certain treatment strategies. Another way is that, as with mutation testing, apolipoprotein E genotyping may become an indicator for prophylactic treatment. A third way is that once the diagnosis of dementia is made, apolipoprotein E genotyping may be of use in further differentiation to diagnose Alzheimer's disease.

CONCLUSION

Alzheimer's disease is being investigated in a multidisciplinary effort. As technological advances are made, our understanding of the disease increases. Molecular genetic approaches in Alzheimer's disease simply were not possible in the mid-1970s. Similarly, advances in neuroradiology and neuropharmacology are reflected in the studies presented. In terms of etiology clearly genetic factors interact with the aging process to trigger the disease. Many other mechanisms may temper this process, such as those associated with gender differences, inflammatory processes, or environmental factors such as head injury. These factors may be of importance in regulating the rate of disease progression. Therefore, beneficial effects may be obtained from therapeutic strategies that have an impact on these mechanisms. However, the goal of basic research is to understand the fundamental etiology of Alzheimer's disease. At that point radical preventive therapies will be possible. It remains to be seen whether such strategies can realistically be employed.

REFERENCES

Alzheimer, A. (1906). Uber Einen Eigenartigen Schweren Krankheitsprozess der Hirnrinde. *Zentralblatt fuer Nervenknankenhaus, 25,* 1134.

Alzheimer, A. (1907a). Uber Eine Eigenartige Erkrankung der Hirnrinde. *Allgemeine Zeitschrift fuer Psychiatrie, 64,* 146.

Alzheimer, A. (1907b). Uber Einen Eigenartigen Schweren Krankenheitsprozess der Hirnrinde. *Zentralblatt fuer Nervenknankenhaus, 30,* 177.

Amaducci, L.A., Fratiglioni, L., Rocca, W.A., Fieschi, C., Livrea, P., Pedone, D., Bracco, L., Lippi, A., Gandolfo, C., & Bino, G. (1986). Risk factors for clinically diagnosed Alzheimer's disease: A case-control study of an Italian population. *Neurology, 36*(7), 922–931.

American Psychiatric Association. (1994). *The diagnostic and statistical manual of mental disorders* (4th ed.), Washington, DC: Author.

Bartus, R.T., Dean, R.L., Beer, B., & Lippa, A.S. (1982). The cholinergic hypothesis of geriatric memory dysfunction. *Science, 217,* 408–417.

Beerman, B. (1993). Side effects of long-acting cholinesterase inhibitors. *Acta Neurologica Scandinavica (Supplement), 149,* 53–54.

Bennett, C., Crawford, F., Osborne, A., Diaz, P., Hoyne, J., Lopez, R., Roques, P., Duara, R., Rossor, M., & Mullan, M. (1995). Evidence that the APOE locus influences rate of disease progression in late onset familial Alzheimer's disease but is not causative. *American Journal of Medical Genetics (Neuropsychiatric Genetics), 60,* 1–6.

Bohnen, N., Warner, M., Kokmen, E., Beard, C., & Kurland, L. (1994). Alzheimer's disease and cumulative exposure to anesthesia: A case-control study. *Journal of the American Geriatric Society, 42,* 198–201.

Breitner, J., Gau, B., Welsh, K., Plassman, B., McDonald, W., Helms, M., & Anthony, J. (1994). Inverse association of anti-inflammatory treatments and Alzheimer's disease: Initial results of a co-twin control study. *Neurology, 44*(2), 227–232.

Breteler, M.M., Claus, J.J., van Duijn, C.M., Launer, L.J., & Hofman, A. (1992). Epidemiology of Alzheimer's disease. *Epidemiologic Reviews, 14,* 59–82.

Broe, G.A., Henderson, A.S., Creasey, H., McCusker, E., Korten, A.E., Jorm, A.F., Longley, W., & Anthony, J.C. (1990). A case-control study of Alzheimer's disease in Australia. *Neurology, 40*(11), 1698–1707.

Chandra, V., Kokmen, E., Schoenberg, B.S., & Beard, C.M. (1989). Head trauma with loss of consciousness as a risk factor for Alzheimer's disease. *Neurology, 39*(12), 1576–1578.

Chartier-Harlin, M.C., Crawford, F., Houlden, H., Warren, A., Hughes, D., Fidani, L., Goate, A., Rossor, M., Roques, P., & Hardy, J. (1991). Early onset Alzheimer's disease caused by mutations at codon 717 of the β-amyloid precursor protein gene. *Nature, 353,* 844–846.

Chatellier, G., & Lacomblez, L. (1990). Tacrine and lecithin in senile dementia of the Alzheimer type: A multicentre trial. *British Medical Journal, 300*, 495–499.

Coyle, J.T., Price, D.L., & DeLong, M.R. (1983). Alzheimer's disease: A disorder of cortical cholinergic innervation. *Science, 219*(4589), 1184–1190.

Dartigues, J.F., Gagnon, M., Barberger-Gateau, P., Letenneur, L., Commenges, D., Sauvel, C., Michel, P., & Salamon, R. (1992). The paquid epidemiological program on brain ageing. *Neuroepidemiology, 11*(suppl. 1), 1–122.

Davis, K.L., Thal, L.J., Gamzu, E.R., Davis, C.S., Woolson, R.F., Gracon, S.I., Drachman, D.A., Schneider, L.S., Whitehouse, P.J., & Hoover, T.M. (1992). A double-blind, placebo-controlled multicenter study of tacrine for Alzheimer's disease. *New England Journal of Medicine, 327*(18), 1253–1259.

Delaere, P., Duyckaerts, C., Masters, C., Beyreuther, K., Piette, F., & Hauw, J.J. (1990). Large amounts of neocortical beta A4 deposits without neuritic plaques nor tangles in a psychometrically assessed, non-demented person. *Neuroscience Letters, 116*(1–2), 87–93.

Diesfeldt, H.F., van Houte, L.R., & Moerkens, R.M. (1986). Duration and survival in senile dementia. *Acta Psychiatrica Scandinavica, 73*, 366–371.

Dunnett, S.B., & Fibiger, H.C. (1993). Role of forebrain cholinergic systems in learning and memory: Relevance to the cognitive deficits of aging and AD dementia. *Progress in Brain Research, 98*, 413–420.

Eagger, S.A., Levy, R., & Sahakian, B.J. (1991). Tacrine in Alzheimer's disease. *Lancet, 337*, 989–992.

Enz, A., Amstutz, R., Boddeke, H., Gmelin, G., & Malanowski, J. (1993). Brain selective inhibition of acetylcholinesterase: A novel approach to therapy for Alzheimer's disease. *Progress in Brain Research, 98*, 431–438.

Ernst, R., & Hay, J. (1994). The U.S. economic and social costs of Alzheimer's disease revisited. *American Journal of Public Health, 84*, 1261–1264.

Fischer, W., Wictorin, K., Bjorklund, A., Williams, L.R., Varon, S., & Gage, F.H. (1987). Amelioration of cholinergic neuron atrophy and spatial memory impairment in aged rats by nerve growth factor. *Nature, 329*, 65–68.

Foncin, J. (1987). Alzheimer's disease and aluminum [letter]. *Nature, 326*, 136.

Fratiglioni, L. (1993). Epidemiology of Alzheimer's disease: Issues of etiology and validity. *Acta Psychiatrica Scandinavica, 143*(suppl.), 1–70.

Gauthier, S., Bouchard, R., Lamontagne, A., Bailey, P., & Bergman, H. (1990). Tetrahydroaminoacridine-lecithin combination treatment in patients with intermediate-stage Alzheimer's disease. *New England Journal of Medicine, 322*, 1272–1276.

Giacobini, E. (1993). Pharmacotherapy of Alzheimer's disease: New drugs and novel strategies. *Progress in Brain Research, 98*, 447–454.

Glenner, C., & Wong, C. (1984). Alzheimer's disease: Initial report of the purification and characterization of a novel cerebrovascular amyloid protein. *Biochemical and Biophysical Research Communication, 120*, 885–890.

Goate, A., Rossor, M., Roques, P., Hardy, J., & Mullan, M. (1991). Segregation of the missense mutation in the amyloid precursor gene with familial Alzheimer's disease. *Nature, 353*, 844–846.

Goldgaber, D., Lerman, M., McBride, W., Saffiotti, U., & Gajdusek, D. (1987). Isolation, characterization, and chromosomal localization of human brain cDNA clones coding for the precursor of the amyloid of brain in Alzheimer's disease, Down's syndrome, and aging. *Journal of Neural Transmission, 24*(suppl.), 23–28.

Graves, A.B., White, E., Koepsell, T.D., Reifler, B.V., van Belle, G., Larson, E.B., & Raskind, M. (1990a). A case-control study of Alzheimer's disease. *Annals of Neurology, 28*(6), 766–774.

Graves, A.B., White, E., Koepsell, T., Reifler, B., van Belle, G., & Larson, E. (1990b). The association between aluminum-containing products and Alzheimer's disease. *Journal of Clinical Epidemiology, 43*(1), 35–44.

Gustafson, L. (1992). Clinical classification of dementia conditions. *Acta Neurologica Scandinavica, 139*(suppl.), 16–20.

Handelman, G., Boyles, J., Weisgraber, K., Mahley, R., & Pitas, R. (1992). Effects of apolipoprotein E, beta-very low density lipoproteins, and cholesterol on other extensions of neurites by rabbit dorsal root ganglio neurons *in vivo*. *Journal of Lipid Research, 33*(11), 1677–1688.

Henderson, V., Paganini-Hill, A., Emanuel, C.K., Dunn, M.E., & Buckwalter, J.G. (1994). Estrogen replacement therapy in older women. Comparisons between Alzheimer's disease cases and non-demented control subjects. *Archives of Neurology, 51*(9), 896–900.

Heyman, A., Wilkinson, W., & Hurwitz, B. (1987). Early-onset Alzheimer's disease: Clinical predictors of institutionalization and death. *Neurology, 38*, 975–980.

Honjo, H., Tamura, T., Matsumoto, Y., Kawata, M., Ogino, Y., Tanaka, K., Yamamoto, T., Ueda, S., & Okada, H. (1992). Estrogen as a growth factor to central nervous cells. Estrogen treatment promotes development of acetylcholinesterase positive basal forebrain neurons transplanted in the anterior eye chamber. *Journal of Steroid Biochemistry and Molecular Biology, 41*(3–8), 633–635.

Jones, M.J. (1989). The influence of anesthetic methods on mental function. *Acta Chirurgica Scandinavica, 550*(suppl.), 169–175.

Jorm, A. (1991). Cross-national comparisons of the occurrence of Alzheimer's and vascular dementias. *European Archives of Psychiatry and Clinical Neuroscience, 240*, 218–222.

Jorm, A., Dorten, A., & Henderson, A. (1987). The prevalence of dementia: A quantitative integration of the literature. *Acta Psychiatrica Scandinavica, 76*, 465–479.

Kamboh, M.I., Sanghera, D.K., Ferrell, R., & DeKosky, S.T. (1995). APOE*4-associated Alzheimer's disease risk is modified by alpha 1-antichymotrypsin polymorphism. *Nature Genetics, 10*, 486–488.

Katzman, R., & Thal, L. (1989). Neurochemistry of Alzheimer's disease. In G.J. Siegel (Ed.), *Basic neurochemistry: Molecular, cellular, and medical aspects* (5th ed., p. 1104). New York: Raven Press.

Kokmen, E., Beard, C., & Offord, K. (1989). Prevalence of medically diagnosed dementia in a defined United States population: Rochester, Minnesota, January 1, 1975. *Neurology, 39*, 773–776.

Kokmen, E., Chandra, V., & Schoenberg, B. (1988). Trends in incidence of dementing illness in Rochester, Minnesota, in three quinquennial periods, 1960–1974. *Neurology, 38*, 975–980.

Lannfelt, L., Lilius, L., Appelgren, H., Axelman, K., Forsell, C., Liu, L., Johansson, K., & Graff, C. (1993). No linkage to chromosome 14 in Swedish Alzheimer's disease families [letter]. *Nature Genetics, 4*, 218–219.

Levy-Lahad, E., Wasco, W., Poorkaj, P., Romano, D., Oshima, J., Pettingell, W., Yu, C., Jondro, P., Schmidt, S., Wang, K., Crowley, A., Fu, Y., Guenette, S., Galas, D., Nemems, E., Wijsman, E., Bird, T., Schellenberg, G., & Tanzi, R. (1995). Candidate gene for the chromosome 1 familial Alzheimer's disease locus. *Science, 269*, 973–977.

Li, G., Shen, Y.C., Chen, C.H., Zhau, Y.W., & Silverman, J.M. (1992). A case-control study of Alzheimer's disease in China. *Neurology, 42*(8), 1481–1488.

Martyn, C., & Barker, D. (1989). Geographical relation between Alzheimer's disease and aluminum in drinking water. *Lancet, 1*, 59–62.

McGeer, P., Akiyama, H., Itagaki, S., & McGeer, E. (1989). Immune system response in Alzheimer's disease. *Canadian Journal of Neurological Science, 16*, 516–527.

McKhann, G., Drachman, D., Folstein, M., Katzman, R., Price, D., & Stadlan, E.M. (1984). Clinical diagnosis of Alzheimer's disease: Report of the NINCDS-ADRA work group under the auspices of Department of Health and Human Services Task Force on Alzheimer's Disease. *Neurology, 34*, 939–944.

Molloy, D.W., Guyatt, G.H., Wilson, D.B., Duke, R., Rees, L., & Singer, J. (1991). Effect of tetrahydroaminoacridine on cognition, function, and behavior in Alzheimer's disease. *Canadian Medical Association Journal, 144*, 29–34.

Mullan, M., Bennett, C., Figueredo, C., Hughes, D., Mant, R., Owen, M., Warren, A., McInnis, M., Marshall, A., Lantos, P., Collinge, J., Goate, A., Houlden, H., & Crawford, C. (1994). Clinical features of early onset, familial Alzheimer's disease linked to chromosome 14. *American Journal of Medical Genetics (Neuropsychiatric Genetics), 60*, 44–52.

Mullan, M., & Brown, J. (1994). The clinical features of Alzheimer's disease and the search for clinico-aetiologic correlates. *Anti-Dementia Agents, 1*, 1–12.

Mullan, M., & Crawford, F. (1993). Genetic and molecular advances in Alzheimer's disease. *Trends in Neuroscience, 16*(10), 398–403.

Mullan, M., Houlden, H., Crawford, F., Kennedy, A., Rogues, P., & Rossor, M. (1993). Age of onset in familial early onset Alzheimer's disease correlates with genetic etiology. *American Journal of Medical Genetics (Neuropsychiatric Genetics), 48*, 129–130.

Mullan, M., Houlden, H., Windelspecht, M., Fidani, L., & Lombardi, C. (1992). A locus for familial early-onset Alzheimer's disease on the long arm of chromosome 14, proximal to the alpha-antichymotrypsin gene. *Nature Genetics, 2*, 340–342.

Mulnard, R., Cotman, C., Koff, E., Sano, M., Thal, L., Grundman, M., & Klauber, M. (1995). *A multicenter double-blind placebo-controlled study of estrogen replacement therapy in patients with mild to moderate Alzheimer's disease. A pilot study of the Alzheimer's Disease Cooperative Study Unit (ADCSU)*. Rockville, MD: National Institute on Aging.

Murrell, J., Farlow, M., Ghetti, B., & Benson, M. (1991). A mutation in the amyloid precursor protein associated with hereditary Alzheimer's disease. *Science, 254*, 97–99.

Noguchi, S., Murakaami, K., & Yamada, N. (1993). Apolipoprotein E genotype and Alzheimer's disease [letter]. *Lancet, 342*, 1309.

O'Connor, D., Pollitt, P., & Hyde, J. (1989). The prevalence of dementia as measured by the Cambridge Mental Disorders of the Elderly Examination. *Acta Psychiatrica Scandinavica, 79*, 198–208.

Okuizumi, K., Onodera, O., Namba, Y., Ikeda, K., Yamamoto, T., Seki, K., Ueki, A., Nanko, S., Tanaka, H., Takashi, H., Oyanagi, K., Mizuasawa, H., Kananzawa, I., & Tsuji, S. (1995). Genetic association of the very low density lipoprotein (VLDL) receptor gene with sporadic Alzheimer's disease. *Nature Genetics, 11*, 207–209.

Paganini-Hill, A., & Henderson, V. (1994). Estrogen deficiency and risk of Alzheimer's disease in women. *American Journal of Epidemiology, 140*(3), 256–261.

Poduslo, S.E., Riggs, D., Schwankhaus, J., Mullan, M., Crawford, F., & Osborne, A. (1995). Association of apolipoprotein E but not B with Alzheimer's disease. *Hum Genet, 254*, 1–4.

Porier, J., Davignon, J., Bouthillier, D., Kogan, S., Bertrand, P., & Gauthier, S. (1993). Apolipoprotein E polymorphism and Alzheimer's disease. *Lancet, 342*, 697–699.

Rebeck, G.W., Perls, T.T., West, H.L., Sodhi, P., Lipsitz, L.A., & Hyman, B.T. (1994). Reduced apolipoprotein epsilon 4 allele frequency in the oldest old Alzheimer's patients and cognitively normal individuals. *Neurology, 44*(8), 1513–1516.

Rebeck, G., Reiter, J., Strickland, D., & Hyman, B. (1993). Apolipoprotein in sporadic Alzheimer's disease: Allelic variation and receptor interactions. *Neuron, 11*, 575–580.

Rich, J., Rasmusson, D., Folstein, M., Carson, K., Kawas, C., & Brandt, J. (1995). Nonsteroidal anti-inflammatory drugs in Alzheimer's disease. *Neurology, 45*, 51–55.

Risse, S.C., Lampe, T.H., Bird, T.D., Nochlin, D., Sumi, S.M., Keenan, T., Cubberley, L., Peskind, E., & Raskind, M.A. (1990). Myoclonus, seizures, and paratonia in Alzheimer's disease. *Alzheimer's Disease and Associated Disorders, 4*(4), 217–225.

Rocca, W., Amaducci, L., & Schoenberg, B. (1986). Epidemiology of clinically diagnosed Alzheimer's disease. *Annals of Neurology, 19*, 415–424.

Rocca, W.A., Bonaiuto, S., Lippi, A., Luciani, P., Turtu, F., Cavarzeran, F., & Amaducci, L. (1990). Prevalence of clinically diagnosed Alzheimer's disease and other dementing disorders: A door-to-door survey in Appignano, Macerata Province, Italy. *Neurology, 40*(4), 626–631.

Rocca, W.A., Hofman, A., Brayne, C., Breteler, M., Clarke, M., Copeland, J., Dartigues, J.F., Engedal, K., Hagnell, O., Heeren, T., Jonker, C., Lindesay, J., Lobo, A., Mann, A., Molsa, P., Morgan, K., O'Connor, D., Silva Droux, A., Sulkava, R., Kay, D., & Amaducci, L. (1991). The prevalence of vascular dementia in Europe: Facts and fragments from 1980–1990 studies. *Annals of Neurology, 30*(6), 817–824.

Rogers, J., Kirby, L.C., Hempelman, S.R., Berry, D.L., McGeer, P.L., Kaszniak, A.W., Zalinski, J., Cofield, M., Mansukhani, L., Willson, P., & Kogan, F. (1993). Clinical trial of indomethacin in Alzheimer's disease. *Neurology, 43*, 1609–1611.

Rorsman, B., Hagnell, O., & Lanke, J. (1986). Prevalence and incidence of senile and multi-farct dementia in the Lundby study: A comparison between the time periods 1947–1957 and 1957–1972. *Neuropsychobiology, 15*, 122–129.

Schellenberg, G.D., Bird, T.D., Wijsman, E.M., Moore, D.K., Boehnke, M., Bryant, E.M., Lampe, T.H., Nochlin, D., Sumi, S.M., & Deeb, J.J. (1988). Absence of linkage of chromosome 21q21 markers to familial Alzheimer's disease. *Science, 241*(4872), 1507–1510.

Schellenberg, G.D., Bird, T.D., Wijsman, E.M., Orr, H.T., Anderson, L., Nemens, E., White, J.A., Bonnycastle, L., Weber, J.L., & Alonso, M.E. (1992). Genetic linkage evidence for a familial Alzheimer's disease locus on chromosome 14. *Science, 258*, 668–671.

Schellenberg, G.D., Deeb, S.S., Boehnke, M., Bryant, E.M., Martin, G.M., Lampe, T.H., & Bird, T.D. (1987). Association of an apolipoprotein CII allele with familial dementia of the Alzheimer type. *Journal of Neurogenetics, 4*(2–3), 97–108.

Schoenberg, B., Kokmen, E., & Okazaki, H. (1987). Alzheimer's disease and other dementing illnesses in a defined United States population: Incidence rates and clinical features. *Annals of Neurology, 22*, 724–729.

Scinto, L., Daffner, K., Dressler, D., Ransil, B., Rentz, D., Weintraub, S., Mesulam, M., & Potter, H. (1994). A potential non-invasive neurobiological test for Alzheimer's disease. *Science, 266*, 1051–1054.

Sobel, E., Louhija, J., Sulkava, R., Davanipour, Z., Kantula, K., Miettinen, H., Tikkanen, M., Kainulainen, K., & Tilvis, R. (1995). Lack of association of apolipoprotein E allele E4 with late-onset Alzheimer's disease among Finnish centenarians. *Neurology, 45*, 903–907.

St. George-Hyslop, P.H., Haines, J.L., & Farrer, L.A. (1990). Genetic linkage studies suggest that Alzheimer's disease is not a single homogeneous disorder (FAD Collaborative Study Group). *Nature, 347*, 194–197.

St. George-Hyslop, P., McLachlan, D., Tsuda, T., Rogaev, E., Karlinsky, H., Lippa, C., & Pollen, D. (1994). Alzheimer's disease and possible gene interaction. *Science, 263*(5146), 537.

Strittmatter, W.J., Saunders, A.M., Schmechel, D., St. George-Hyslop, P.H., Pericak-Vance, M.A., Joo, S.H., Rosi, B.L., Gusella, J.F., Crapper-MacLachlan, D.R., & Alberts, M.J. (1993). Association of apolipoprotein E allele epsilon 4 with late-onset familial and sporadic Alzheimer's disease. *Neurology, 43*(8), 1467–1472.

Tanzi, R., Gusella, J., Watkins, P., Bruns, G., & St. George-Hyslop, P. (1987). Amyloid beta protein gene: cDNA, mRNA distribution, and genetic linkage near the Alzheimer locus. *Science, 235*, 880–884.

Van Broeckhoven, C., Backhovens, H., Cruts, M., Martin, J., Crook, R., Houlden, H., & Hardy, J. (1994). APOE genotype does not modulate age of onset in families with chromosome 14 encoded Alzheimer's disease. *Neuroscience Letters, 169*, 179–180.

van Duijn, C.M., Stijnen, T., & Hofman, A. (1994). Risk factors for Alzheimer's disease: Overview of the EURODERM collaborative re-analysis of case-control studies. *International Journal of Epidemiology, 2*(20 suppl.), S4–S12.

Whitehouse, P.J. (1993). Cholinergic therapy in dementia. *Acta Neurologica Scandinavica, 149*, 42–45.

Wolf-Klein, G.P. (1993). New Alzheimer's drug expands your options in symptom management. *Geriatrics, 48*(8), 26–36.

Zhang, M., Datzman, R., & Salmon, D. (1990). The prevalence of dementia and Alzheimer's disease in Shanghai, China: Impact of age, gender and education. *Annals of Neurology, 27*, 428–437.

11

Innovations in Special Care Programs

Stephanie B. Hoffman, Ph.D.

Units for people who display aberrant behavior are not especially new or innovative. They are as old as the locked wards in state mental hospitals, as prevalent as prisons and jails. Locked dementia-specific care units, with no special programming, no trained staff, and no sense of safety and comfort for residents, are in essence depriving people with dementia of their civil rights. The innovations described in this chapter are features of a special care program that will give meaning and dignity to the lives of people with dementing illnesses. The features are not especially high tech; in fact, the more successful programs are "high touch."

The greatest successes and creative ideas of respondents to the questionnaire distributed at the conference, *Dementia Specific Care Units: Winning Strategies for Success*, are addressed first. Then a review is provided of selected ideas and suggestions submitted to the conference competition. Unusual and creative ideas warranting dissemination were described in a number of these applications.

GREATEST SUCCESSES

Successes in programming and management were described in many responses to the questionnaire. Some respondents felt that mere survival was their greatest success. Others reported receiving additional capital funding. Staff involvement in planning led to success in several programs. One facility was proud of its full occupancy and its good bottom line and reputation, another facility was proud to have been able to establish excellent rapport with residents and families. Design was seen as vital to several programs, especially designs that minimized confusion, lessened noise, utilized features that were family friendly, maintained a restraint-free setting, or educated architects in the needs of residents with dementia. The facility that had successfully educated its architects had street scenes, home fronts on the outside of resident rooms, and hallway alcoves for holding small groups. Several programs developed a partnership for care with families. One setting was proud of its personalized programs. Staff incentives were noticeable, including staff retention programs, training programs for staff and permanent floater personnel, and a ratio of staff to residents that facilitated care.

CREATIVE IDEAS

Innovative training programs for staff were described in several responses to the questionnaire. One facility reported training in patient sexuality. Another facility ran a support group for certified nursing assistants. Several settings emphasized their interdisciplinary teams as a motivating force with staff. The inclusion of a geropsychologist was particularly helpful to one setting, as this discipline conducted neuropsychological assessments and advised on behavior management techniques. A Canadian facility used a psychogeriatric nurse in this role. Training the permanent floater staff was felt to be important, as was involving an ombudsperson to meet with difficult families on a scheduled basis. Another facility introduced a case management system. One successful facility had its non-nursing personnel "adopt a resident." Some respondents reported that technology played a role in certain innovations. Computer-based interdisciplinary care plans with scheduled interventions and flow sheets were particularly useful to them.

Activities were at the heart of several successful programs. One facility ran an activity therapy program 12 hours per day; another program included several activities at night. Some creative group activities for residents included validation therapy, a sundowner's program, adult day services, daily sing-along with song sheets, a creative dance movement class, the "poet's society," a passive range of motion class, an ambulation program, and music therapy. The use of music, art, humor, and tactile therapy was important to many facilities. One creative idea was a "Fuss and Flatter" morning program that involved residents in their personal grooming.

One program established a work program to give residents a feeling of worth.

Approaches to nutrition programs were creative in some facilities. One setting used bulk food service instead of tray service. In a "Silver Spoons" feeding program, older people without cognitive impairment were asked to assist residents with feeding. Occupational therapy ran a resource dining program in several places.

Volunteers were incorporated into the programming by several facilities. In one facility community activities, such as fishing or going out to eat in a restaurant in the community, were encouraged once a month.

Respecting the rights of residents was emphasized by some facilities. One facility permitted all residents to stay in bed until they awakened on their own. Another facility wanted residents to be as restraint free as possible. The ability to allow residents to die with dignity was encouraged in a hospice-type facility.

SPECIFIC INNOVATIVE SUBMISSIONS

The following programs and ideas were submitted to the conference. They are innovative, unusual, and exciting suggestions for improving the quality of life of people with dementia.

Music Therapy

The Vestal (New York) Nursing Center (Johnson, 1995) conducts a music therapy program with residents with severe dementia, funded as a research project by the New York State Department of Health to examine the effect of music therapy on agitation and cognition. Each resident at the center receives two small group music therapy sessions and one individual music therapy session per week. Validation and redirection through music are emphasized. Residents' emotions are validated through permission to express emotions with songs or emotional playing of musical instruments. Rhythm and tempo can match their repetitive movements and pacing. Redirection occurs when music is used to change moods or to provide comfort and relaxation, which can interrupt a perseverative (repetition beyond a desired point) pattern. A variety of remembered and new skills, sensory stimulation, reminiscence, comfort, and renewed communication are outcomes of this experience.

Design Features that Increase Autonomy

The Corinne Dolan Alzheimer Care and Applied Research Center (Chardon, Ohio) has conducted many studies to analyze the impact of design features on resident autonomy (Harr, 1995). In particular, staff have noticed that certain environmental features, such as visible toilets, can support toileting skills. The staff has simplified the dressing process to encourage independent dressing. Independent access to outdoor areas also has positive implications for behavior management.

The staff at Hanover Terrace (Hanover, New Hampshire) (Sacco, 1995) developed several meal programs for residents. Residents with mild to moderate dementia are included in a program called Enhanced Dining, in which they set their own tables. Special meal place cards are used for residents who need cuing, with setup instructions on the back of each person's card. Snacks on wheels include foods such as bananas, toast with peanut butter, and high-calorie pudding in plastic mugs. The finger food menu is used with residents who have difficulty with utensils. Finger foods have increased food consumption and decreased residents' frustration.

Normalizing Activities

The Group Home at Foxwood Springs Living Center (Raymore, Missouri) encourages its women residents in activities such as setting and clearing the table for meals, planning menus, shopping for food items, sorting and folding laundry, dusting furniture, and sweeping floors (Wurth, 1995). The program also includes intergenerational activities. Children from a child development center visit weekly for reading and snack time with the residents.

The Jewish Home and Hospital for the Aged (Bronx, New York) (Nicholson, Reshen, Marchello, & Shelkey, 1995) incorporates a fireplace and rocking chairs to create a homelike setting.

The Jewish Home of Central New York (Syracuse) is designing a special "Americana Room" (Bloodgood, 1995). The archives departments of several companies have contributed wall hangings with original magazine advertisements, videos of classic movies, recordings of swing and big band music, and furniture from the 1930s and 1940s. Interviews with each resident ensure that the room contains a personally meaningful item, picture, music, texture, or food for reminiscing and control of agitated behavior (Figure 11.1).

Cole (1995) developed a program called "Stirring Up Memories," which uses foods to provide pleasure and stimulate the senses. Participants examine recipes and ingredients and either cook or watch a demonstration of cooking.

Medication Administration

Because dementia causes some residents to be unable or unwilling to take medications, researchers and practitioners from the University of Tennessee College of Nursing and the Memphis Jewish Home devised an approach that involved a cooperative effort (Hartig, 1995). A multidisciplinary team comprising licensed nurses, a family nurse practitioner, an activity director, and a staff pharmacist was established. This team identified characteristics of resident behavior and situations that caused residents to either accept or refuse medication. They then developed a resident information form with individualized guidelines for administering medications, a description of resident behavior related to medication, and options for handling initial refusal of the medication.

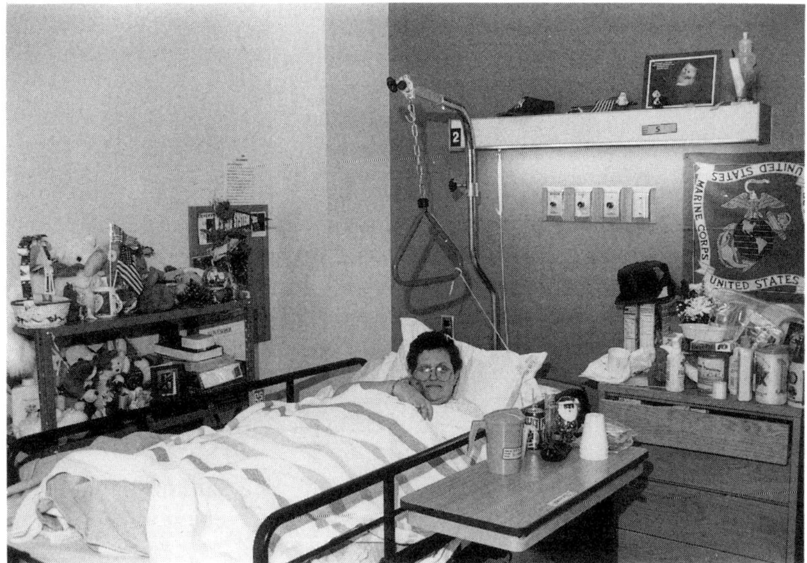

Figure 11.1. This resident personalized her room with mementos and gifts from friends and relatives.

Family Involvement in Care: Family–Staff Partnerships

The Family Involvement in Care program, designed by researchers at the University of Iowa College of Nursing (Maas, 1995), is a staff/family conference for negotiating the type and amount of family involvement in care. Staff and family decide on ways to work together in providing care for the resident with Alzheimer's disease. They then sign a contract to this effect. The staff and family questionnaires developed for evaluating this project may be beneficial to administrators for improving both family satisfaction and efforts toward quality improvement.

Vacation

A 3-day overnight camping trip ("On the Water's Edge") has been developed by an educator/practitioner from Michigan (Ross, 1995). The vacation program has been conducted annually since 1991 and has benefitted 125 older adults and 100 staff and volunteers. The vacation program was created to stimulate the social, interpersonal, and motor skills retained by nursing facility residents with dementia. Residents and facility staff travel by bus from their facilities to a lakeshore campground. Activities during the vacation include marshmallow roasts, campfire singalongs, walks on the beach, and productive tasks at the camp.

Behavioral Treatments

The Geriatric Psychiatry Program of the Medical University of South Carolina (Mintzer et al., 1995) developed a Behavioral Intensive Care Unit program that included several components: thorough in-home evaluation of agitated behaviors and their triggers; interview with the primary physician; a 5-day admission for observation and behavior mapping to identify what causes, maintains, and extinguishes the agitated behaviors; and design and implementation of resident and environmental intervention strategies. Modification of the home environment and training for the primary caregiver are also offered. Agitation was significantly reduced in two thirds of the residents in the program; three fourths of the residents were discharged to their own homes.

Individualized efforts to reduce problem behaviors were tested by Foley and her colleagues and students at Regis College in Weston, Massachusetts (Foley & Ford, 1995). Nonverbal skills used by staff while preparing residents for bed demonstrated a significant decrease in patient agitation. One resident who screamed in the evening responded to 30 minutes of music through headphones and use of chewing gum and writing materials. This resident stopped screaming.

At Rush University in Chicago, Taft (1995) used naturalistic inquiry to develop seven approaches for caregivers when intervening in problem behaviors, including social, psychological, functional, behavioral, environmental, medical, and cognitive approaches. Social approaches were used the most by adult day services staff and included providing activities, relating, empathic caring, and supportive touch. Caregivers used this approach in supporting the personal strengths of the people with dementia for whom they cared.

Mathews (1995), from the University of Kansas, studied the impact of staff training in nine behaviors designed to promote independence of residents in a special care unit. Staff were taught to do the following:

1. Knock on the door before entering the resident's room.
2. Greet the resident by name.
3. Introduce him- or herself to the resident.
4. Create a quiet area with adequate supplies.
5. Clearly specify the task to the resident.
6. Use at least two prompts before using physical guidance.
7. Wait 5–10 seconds between each prompt to give the resident enough time to respond.
8. Use physical guidance correctly.
9. Praise the resident within 5 seconds of successful completion of a task.

Staff significantly increased their performance of these behaviors after the intensive training program and practice sessions.

A unique volunteer program (Keefe, Marvel, & Bermingham, 1995) was developed to examine the effects of using trained volunteers to eliminate or decrease the use of physical and chemical restraints in hospitalized patients with dementia. The volunteers used specialized calming techniques and communication skills to decrease patient agitation. They also collected data for 72 hours using a checklist to assess the number of nurse–patient contacts, use of restraints, and incidence of falls and pulled out tubes.

Sundowner's Program

The Joseph L. Morse Geriatric Center (West Palm Beach, Florida) (Fletcher-Lancto, 1995) runs a daily program from 2:00 to 5:30 P.M. The activities include grooming, toileting, exercise, a tea party, an outdoor stroll, and "fun time." Residents experienced improvements in appetite and sleep; decreased use of antipsychotic drugs; and fewer episodes of wandering, public disrobing, and catastrophes.

Garden of Arden

The Arden Hill Life Care Center (Goshen, New York) (Gallivan & Hopkins, 1995) has a specially designed outdoor garden with wheelchair-accessible planting beds that encourage planting, watering, weeding, and harvesting. The landscape includes walking paths, strawberry patches, herb gardens, and fruit trees. Sitting areas among the many birdhouses offer natural views. A fruit orchard with removable artificial fruit allows for repeated picking of fruit. A wheelchair-accessible sandbox area is also available for feeling, pouring, and molding warm sand. A "traveling garden" on wheels is used for room visits. Volunteers from area garden clubs, master gardeners, and youth from schools and 4-H clubs visit to assist with gardening activities.

Day Services Programs within Nursing Facilities

The Jewish Geriatric Home (Cherry Hill, New Jersey), has created an intensive Safe Haven day services program from 9:00 A.M.–3:00 P.M. for its residents who are depressed or agitated or exhibit socially inappropriate behavior (Adelsberg & Schwartz, 1995). The residents are mainstreamed in the nursing facility during other hours. Activities, including lunch and baking, are held in a large, homey room. The participants are also taken for walks in the facility courtyard. Many classes and therapeutic activities are offered. A similar concept is employed in the Van Duyn Home and Hospital (Syracuse, New York) (Przewlocki, 1995). Van Duyn's Enhanced Activity Program is an 8-hour day that emphasizes a soothing, restraint-free atmosphere. A staff:resident ratio of 1:4 allows significant staff assistance with programs and activities of daily living (ADLs).

A shorter program, The Living Room, is run for 4 hours a day at the Dumont Masonic Home (New Rochelle, New York) (Fetonti, 1995). This program, held from 10:00 A.M. to 2:00 P.M., provides respite for residents without dementia from the inappropriate behaviors of those with dementia.

A family respite center was developed (Handwerk & Noyes, 1995) at Arleigh Burke Pavilion (McLean, Virginia). The program blends day services with assisted living and involves families and residents with mid-stage dementia. One exciting feature is their "Sweet Baby Rounds," in which supervised residents play with and feed babies.

Holiday Survival

Heartland of Perrysburg (Ohio) (Ritter, 1995) has improved the holidays of its dementia-specific care program residents. Staff assist residents in baking treats that can be served to families and exchanged as gifts. Christmas cards with residents' pictures are sent to families. Carolers are encouraged to sing at the Christmas holidays and throughout the year. The sadness and agitation exhibited by residents has been greatly relieved by this approach. Staff at Heartland are encouraged to take photographs of residents to share with families and throughout the facility. These photographs reassure family that their loved ones are participating in enjoyable activities.

Use of Hospice

Simard-Taggart (1994) encourages the use of a hospice for residents within 6 months of death from dementia or accompanying disease. Hospice supports the resident, family, and even the staff and continues to support the family and staff for up to 1 year after the death of the resident. Hospice benefits include medical supplies, durable medical equipment, medications related to the terminal illness, additional nursing assistants, social work services, volunteers to assist the family, and visits from clergy.

Simard-Taggart suggests several indicators for death within 6 months in people with dementia: inability to speak and walk, maximum assistance with ADLs, lack of bladder and bowel control, presence of other life-threatening illnesses, a score of 3 or less on the Mini-Mental State Examination, fever or infection within the last 6 months, and loss of appetite. Smith (1995), at the Geriatric Research, Education and Clinical Centers Dementia Study Units of the Edith Nourse Rogers Memorial Veterans Hospital (Bedford, Massachusetts), includes signs of approaching death within 1 month: a "shutting down," lack of interest in nourishment, and individualized changes in body systems, often with no signs of discomfort. For people in pain, Smith suggests small to moderate doses of morphine or other medications. The hospice approach of the Bedford Veterans Hospital emphasizes providing comfort and dignity to patients, family, and staff.

Staff Training Programs

The education program at the Hebrew Home for the Aged (Riverdale, New York) incorporates diversity training for its staff (Richardson, 1995). Almost every staff member is of an ethnic origin different from that of the residents. The program has four objectives: developing respect for diversity perception, understanding the power of words, identifying differences in nonverbal communication among cultures, and managing behavior.

Chicago's Rush Alzheimer's Disease Center (Hellen, 1995) provides sensitivity training in the intimacy needs of residents. Hellen employs a game called "What Now?" to deal with staff anxiety and increase their skills in managing crises. She also utilizes a preadmission Intimacy Profile and a LifeStory Book.

The Geriatric Department at Parkland Hospital (Dallas, Texas) (Hunley, 1995) provides several hours of free training to home health agency staff, particularly home health aides. Their training emphasizes care issues and behavior management to enhance continuity of care. This group has also developed a simple, basic dementia education manual for families and care providers.

A project to train teenagers in dementia care was launched by Menorah Manor (St. Petersburg, Florida) (Kaplan & Parr, 1995). Developed in collaboration with the Alzheimer's Association Tampa Bay Chapter and the University of South Florida (Tampa) and funded through a grant from the Juvenile Welfare Board, the program used classroom instruction and a practicum of direct interaction with residents of Menorah Manor's 40-bed dementia unit. Following the program, the teenagers involved reported an increase in their knowledge of dementia and the appropriate ways to interact with people with dementia, as well as changes in their attitudes toward people with dementia and older people in general. In addition, positive effects, such as a decrease in problem behaviors and improved mood and affect, were noted in residents with dementia who participated in the program. The teenagers received community service credit for their participation, which met their school and community youth requirements.

Multidimensional Approach

The 520-bed Cobble Hill Nursing Home (Brooklyn, New York) created an Alzheimer's Resource Center to deal with their residents with dementia (Yang-Lewis, 1995), comprising more than 50% of the total population. Their center consists of two 40-bed special care programs, one 40-bed advanced care unit for late-stage residents, three on-unit recreational cluster programs, two off-unit recreational cluster programs, and an interdisciplinary Alzheimer's treatment team. Although staff have clear disciplinary responsibilities, a blurring of roles was also emphasized to gain flexibility and efficiency. Their nursing assistants and recreational therapists conduct activity programs, the recreational therapists assist with certain ADLs, and housekeepers are trained to offer some behavioral interventions. Residents are offered choices in their selection of activities.

CONCLUSIONS

Given that most residents of nursing facilities experience cognitive and/or behavioral problems, it is unfortunate that the innovations described in this chapter are limited to small programs within facilities. It might be more efficacious to implement these programs throughout an entire facility and to develop a small program for people without dementia with its own higher-level programming. Expanding the space and opportunities of nursing facility residents by ensuring that the staff is well trained and the facility is safe and has excellent programming would also greatly enhance their quality of life.

REFERENCES

Adelsberg, R., & Schwartz, J. (1995). *Safe haven* [Abstract]. Jewish Geriatric Home, 3025 West Chapel Avenue, Cherry Hill, NJ 08002.

Bloodgood, M.E. (1995). *Americana therapy* [Abstract]. Jewish Home of Central New York, 4101 East Genessee Street, Syracuse, NY 13214.

Cole, P.J. (1995). *Stirring up memories: Food programs with older adults* [Abstract]. 6595 Fariland Road, Clinton, OH 44216.

Fetonti, L. (1995). *The Living Room: A respite for residents in long term care* [Abstract]. Dumont Masonic Home, 676 Pelham Road, New Rochelle, NY 10805.

Fletcher-Lancto, C. (1995). *Sundowners program for dementia* [Abstract]. Joseph L. Morse Geriatric Center. 4847 Fred Gladstone Drive, West Palm Beach, FL 33417.

Foley, M.E., & Ford, S. (1995). *Pacing, withdrawal, repetitive questions, and screaming in a special care unit: Undergraduate pilot studies to assess behavioral interventions with Alzheimer's residents* [Abstract]. Department of Psychology, Regis College, 235 Wellesley Street, Weston, MA 02193.

Gallivan, M.J., & Hopkins, M.A. (1995). *Pianos, peaches, and pines: Peaceful partnerships and compassionate environments for residents with Alzheimer's disease and related disorders* [Abstract]. Arden Hill Life Care Center, 6 Harriman Drive, Goshen, NY 10924.

Handwerk, L., & Noyes, L.E. (1995). *The best of both worlds: Blending daycare programming with assisted living for people with dementia* [Abstract]. Family Respite Center, 1739 Kirby Road, McLean, VA 22101.

Harr, R.G. (1995). *Applied research design studies that enhance the environmental and programmatic autonomy for those suffering from Alzheimer's disease* [Abstract]. Heather Hill, 12340 Bass Lake Road, Chardon, OH 44024-9364.

Hartig, M.T. (1995). *Medication administration for nursing home residents with dementia: Challenges and success* [Abstract]. University of Tennessee, College of Nursing, 877 Madison Avenue, Memphis, TN 38163.

Hellen, C.R. (1995). *Dementia and expressions of intimacy: specific care unit issues and staff training* [Abstract]. Rush Alzheimer's Disease Center, 710 South Paulina Street, Chicago, IL 60612-3872.

Hunley, J. (1995). *Development of a dementia education manual and subsequent home health agency training* [Abstract]. Department of Geriatrics, Parkland Memorial Hospital, 5201 Harry Hines Boulevard, Dallas, TX 75235.

Johnson, D.B. (1995). *Music therapy dementia programming* [Abstract]. Vestal Nursing Center, 860 Old Vestal Road, Vestal, NY 13850.

Kaplan, M., & Parr, J. (1995). *Teen training in dementia care project.* Paper presented at the Gerontological Society of America meeting, Los Angeles.

Keefe, M., Marvel, K., & Bermingham, R. (1995). *The VITAL Project: Volunteer intervention, training, and advocacy link* [Abstract]. Poudre Valley Hospital, Family Medicine Residency Program, 1025 Pennock Place, Fort Collins, CO 80524.

Maas, M. (1995). *Family involvement in care: Family-staff partnerships* [Abstract]. College of Nursing, University of Iowa, Iowa City, Iowa 52242.

Mathews, R.M. (1995). *Promoting independence in residents of an Alzheimer's special care unit* [Abstract]. Gerontology Center, University of Kansas, Lawrence, KS 66045.

Mintzer, J.E., Lewis, L., Pennypaker, L., Simpson, W., Bachman, D., Huggins, E., Wohlreich, G., Meeks, A., Hunt, S., & Sampson, R. (1995). *Behavioral intensive care unit: A new concept in the management of acute agitated behavior in elderly demented patients* [Abstract]. Geriatric Psychiatry Program, Medical University of South Carolina, Institute of Psychiatry PH141, 171 Ashley Avenue, Charleston, SC 29425.

Nicholson, J., Reshen, A.B., Marchello, V., & Shelkey, M. (1995). *Do rocking chairs by a fireplace make a difference? The interaction of environmental design and therapeutic interventions in specialized Alzheimer's care* [Abstract]. Jewish Home and Hospital for Aged—Bronx Division, 100 West Kingsbridge Road, Bronx, NY 10468.

Przewlocki, A. (1995). *Enhanced activity program: Winning strategy for success* [Abstract]. Van Duyn Home and Hospital, 5075 West Seneca Turnpike, Syracuse, NY 13215.

Richardson, M.B. (1995). *Multicultural communication skills for working with dementia residents* [Abstract]. Hebrew Home for the Aged at Riverdale/Palisade Nursing Home, 5901 Palisade Avenue, Riverdale, NY 10471.

Ritter, L. (1995). *Surviving the holidays in an Alzheimer's special care unit* [Abstract]. Heartland of Perrysburg, 10540 Fremont Pike, Perrysburg, OH 43551.

Ross, K. (1995). *On the water's edge: A vacation for older adults with dementia* [Abstract]. Department of Gerontology, Madonna University, 36600 Schoolcraft Road, Livonia, MI 48150.

Sacco, M. (1995). *Chez Hanover Terrace: A unique dining experience on an Alzheimer's unit* [Abstract]. Hanover Terrace Healthcare, Lyme Road, Hanover, NH 03755.

Simard-Taggart, J. (1994, August). Hospice lends a hand. *Provider, 20,* 41–42.

Smith, S.J. (1995). *Providing comfort to the Alzheimer patient in the dying process* [Abstract]. GRECC Dementia Study Units, Edith Nourse Rogers Memorial Veterans Hospital, Bedford, MA 01730.

Taft, L.B. (1995). *Dementia care: Interventions and factors influencing caregiving approaches* [Abstract]. Rush University, Chicago, IL 60612.

Wurth, J. (1995). Foxwood Springs Living Center, Alzheimer's care center group home model (assisted living) [Abstract]. 1500 West Foxwood Drive, P.O. Box 1172, Raymore, MO 64083.

Yang-Lewis, T. (1995). *The Alzheimer's Resource Center: Facing the challenge—meeting the need* [Abstract]. Cobble Hill Nursing Home, 380 Henry Street, Brooklyn, NY 11201.

12

The Future of Special Care Programs

Philip D. Sloane, M.D., M.P.H., and David A. Lindeman, Ph.D.

What is the future of special care programs? Do they represent, as some have speculated, a passing fashion, a concept that will ultimately disappear within a more enlightened, generalist long-term care practice? Or are special care programs a new and better service delivery form, whose future role will be both distinctive and prominent?

Before attempting to answer these questions, this chapter examines three related trends that the authors expect to help shape the future of special care programs: the evolution of specialized Alzheimer's disease care, the anticipated growth of the number of people with Alzheimer's disease and of their service needs, and developments in the U.S. health care system.

THE HISTORY OF SPECIALIZED DEMENTIA CARE

Specialized institutional care for people with dementia has evolved through several distinct stages (Table 12.1). Initially, dementia-specific units were modeled after wards in mental hospitals. Over time, specialization was extended to include a number of approaches and settings. With

Table 12.1. Stages in development of special care programs

Years	Emphasis	Features
1960–1983	Psychiatry	Most units in large, nonprofit facilities Units modeled after psychiatric wards Placement based largely on behavior Widespread use of physical and pharmacological restraints
1983–1990	Activities and marketing	Proliferation of units in for-profit nursing facilities Units targeted toward early and mid-stage dementia Focus on activities, homelike atmosphere, and minimal use of restraints
1990–	Diversification	Rapid growth of specialization in residential care and adult day services Emphasis on continuum of care for people with dementia Increased specialization and professionalization of staff Heightened competition

the growth of specialized settings has come the development of new professional fields focusing on dementia care.

Earliest Units: The Psychiatric Ward Model

The earliest dementia-specific units arose in large nonprofit nursing facilities. These facilities often housed several hundred residents, including some who were extremely disruptive behaviorally. To make the other wards more peaceful and to try to better serve these difficult residents, some facilities began congregating individuals with dementia in behavioral units.

The model was the inpatient psychiatric ward, and indeed these units often had psychiatrists as medical directors. Two types of people with dementia tended to be placed in these early segregated units: 1) people with early or mid-stage dementia who came into conflict with others by wandering into other people's personal space, taking other people's possessions, starting arguments or fights, or persistently trying to exit the building; and 2) people with late-stage dementia who screamed or hollered or who fought caregivers and (occasionally) other residents. Units were typically locked, and physical and pharmacological restraints were used liberally. The most common activities for the residents of these units were undirected wandering and sitting tied to a chair in front of the nursing station.

Emergence of Activity-Focused Units

During the 1980s, changes in the understanding of dementia were mirrored by the evolution and expansion of specialized dementia care. Central to these changes was the rapid growth of medical knowledge and community awareness about dementia. "Senility" was no longer considered a normal part of aging, but rather a medical problem that should be actively investigated and treated. As the public became more aware of Alzheimer's disease, they became receptive to the idea of specialized services for people with the disease. Thus, the concept of a state-of-the-art special care program for people with dementia was able to catch the fancy of administrators and of marketing departments.

Increased awareness about Alzheimer's disease also led to a growing interest in treating rather than warehousing people with dementia. The strongest influence in this area was Wesley Hall, an 11-bed Alzheimer's unit developed over the years 1983–1985 by Dorothy Coons, a professor of nursing at the University of Michigan (Coons, 1987). The unit was remodeled to be homelike and intimate, and residents were admitted who could participate in group activities. Staff saw themselves as friends and enablers rather than as caregivers. The unit's goals focused on keeping residents involved in tasks that would have meaning, provide pleasure, and utilize the residents' remaining skills. Thus, a program of continuous activities was provided, many of which involved household tasks, such as setting the table, doing laundry, and gardening. Wesley Hall received widespread publicity, and soon a variety of other settings expanded on this work. Corporations such as Hillhaven developed initiatives in specialized care, attempting to find ways to incorporate the principles of more humanistic care to the broader nursing facility industry.

Diversification and Increased Professionalism

By the early 1990s, specialized dementia care was a booming field. No longer was it the sole province of the nursing facility. Instead, special care programs were proliferating in adult day services and residential care (board and care or assisted living settings). Hospice-type programs also began to arise, spurred in part by the pioneering work of Volicer and his colleagues (Volicer, Collard, Hurley, Bishop, Kern, & Karon, 1994). Along with this diversification came an increasing awareness that dementia care needed to be provided along a continuum. In the early stage of the disease a day program focusing on activities might be appropriate. In the mid-stage of the disease a residential program might be most appropriate, with a focus that includes activities, socialization, family involvement, and preservation of mobility, continence, and nutrition. In the late stage of the disease the goals of care might be comfort and nursing, and placement in an end-stage program might be appropriate. In the long-term care industry Manor HealthCare and certain all-dementia facilities, such as the Alois Center and Namaste, have sought to operationalize the concept of a continuum of care for people with dementia.

With this expansion and diversification has come increasing professionalism. Dementia care has become a field with a distinct body of knowledge. Environmental design has evolved tremendously from the naive, simplistic formulas of the late 1980s, such as color coding, which is senseless as an orientation principle because it relies on the ability to abstract, a function that is lost early in Alzheimer's disease. Similarly, therapeutic recreation and activities for people with dementia have emerged as distinct fields, with bodies of knowledge and resource materials that can improve immensely upon what even a creative person can do alone. Finally, nursing and medicine, in concert with rehabilitative disciplines such as physical therapy, have actively sought and developed improved methods of managing dementia. As a result, incontinence can be managed better, immobility delayed, and weight loss prevented, often for years, if state-of-the-art knowledge and skills are available to assist in the planning and provision of care.

ANTICIPATED NEEDS FOR DEMENTIA CARE

Although the sophistication of special dementia care has increased as a result of greater awareness of the disease and improvement in professional care, there is one irrefutable fact: Until a cure is found, the changing demographics of American society indicate that the number of people with Alzheimer's disease will increase. A major shift is occurring as life expectancy increases in the United States, with the proportion of old-old people (age 85 and older) expected to increase by 80% by the year 2000. This growth of the older adult population is and will continue to be accompanied by a concomitant increase in the number of individuals affected by Alzheimer's disease and related dementias. The prevalence of severe dementia among this group may range as high as 45% (Evans, 1990). From 1980 to 2000 the number of people with severe dementia in the United States is projected to grow from 1.4 million to 2.4 million; by 2040 this figure is projected to be 7.3 million (Office of Technology Assessment, 1987).

The probability of nursing facility use also increases sharply with age. Of all people who turned 65 in 1990, 43% are projected to enter a nursing facility at some point before they die, and 21% will have a total lifetime nursing facility use of 5 or more years (Kemper & Murtaugh, 1991). Studies of nursing facility residents indicate that a large and growing percentage have dementia (Lair & Lefkowitz, 1990; U.S. Department of Health and Human Services, 1991). In fact, as many as 78% of nursing facility residents suffer from dementia (Chandler & Chandler, 1988; Rovner, Kalfonek, & Filipp, 1986; Rovner et al., 1990).

Compounding the rising incidence of Alzheimer's disease is the slow, progressive nature of the illness. Its course ranges from a few years to as many as 15 years. In addition, although researchers have identified distinct disease stages, of greater importance is the fact that the progress of the disease is different in each individual, often resulting in unique combinations of behavioral, functional, and cognitive impairments. Thus, the progression of Alzheimer's disease is not always linear and predictable.

Just as the disease varies from person to person over time, individual needs and service requirements vary as people progress through different stages of the disease and as a result of the unique effects of the illness on individuals. In most cases, however, severe impairments ultimately require residential care for an extended period of time. In the early stages of residential care residents often benefit from behavioral management; in the later stages of the disease it is more common for residents to benefit from support for activities of daily living. As knowledge increases regarding ways to deal with specific aspects of dementia, special care programs can be tailored to the individual needs of residents.

The best way to provide care to people with dementia, particularly in residential settings, remains a source of debate. Professionals have been considering the arguments for and against specialized programs for individuals with dementia since the early 1980s. Until the undertaking of systematic research to analyze the outcomes and effectiveness of special care by the National Institute of Aging (Ory, 1994) and other groups, knowledge of the pros and cons of special care programs has been based on very small studies and anecdotal outcomes (Maslow, 1994).

Thus, the impact of special care programs is unclear. As summarized in Table 12.2, many professionals, researchers, and policy makers have suggested that specialized care improves the quality of care and functional level of residents, reducing their excess disabilities and offering individualized plans of care. In addition, it is often posited that the benefits of special care programs extend to residents without dementia by reducing the intrusion and disruption brought by some residents with cognitive impairment; improving family satisfaction; and leading to better trained staff who experience less burnout. Many of these points have yet to be substantiated. In fact, it has often been argued that providing high-quality care to all residents will offer benefits to all individuals requiring nursing care, including residents with dementia. Similarly, being mixed in with individuals without cognitive impairment may help people with dementia, just as improving the ability of all staff to deal with problems associated with dementia can improve the overall quality of staff care.

Although their efficacy has not been proven, special care programs for people with dementia appear to be here to stay. As was true with home care for older people with chronic illness, which grew in spite of controversy over its effectiveness, special care programs are too popular with consumers to do anything but proliferate. The direction of this growth will be determined by changes that occur in the health care system.

Table 12.2. Arguments for and against special programs for people with dementia

Arguments for	Arguments against
The needs of individuals with dementia are not the same as those of individuals who are cognitively intact.	All people need much the same care.
The needs of people with cognitive impairments are different from those of cognitively intact people.	Instead of segregating people, the quality of all care should be upgraded.
Being around people whose mental functioning is higher can be stressful for people with dementia.	Placing people with dementia with people who are cognitively intact helps people with dementia to remain alert.
Special care programs permit special interior design, fire safety equipment, trained staff, and marketing efforts.	Special care programs must hold a bed open until a person with dementia needs it.
Older people who are cognitively intact have often made it clear that they do not want to spend their lives with people with dementia.	In mixed programs individuals who are cognitively intact can help "look after" people with dementia.
The current demand for special care programs is such that family members will transport loved ones with dementia long distances for residential care.	In areas with a low population density there are not enough people with dementia to support special care programs.
An all-dementia program allows staff to develop expertise in caring for residents, often preventing burnout.	Staff will quickly burn out in a special care program.
Residents rights laws, ombudspersons, and quality assurance regulations ensure oversight of people who are not competent.	A program serving people with dementia could create a ghetto in which no one would report abuses or be a legally capable witness.
Dementia is a medical specialty long overdue for recognition.	Dementia is not a medical specialty deserving of separate designation and specialization.

Adapted from Office of Technology Assessment (1987).

THE EVOLVING U.S. HEALTH CARE SYSTEM

As demographics and insights from clinicians and researchers expand special care programs, the programs' specific direction will be greatly influenced by external factors. One of these factors is the major changes that are occurring in the U.S. health care system. Proposed government changes in long-term care in the early 1990s, including the catastrophic Medicare program and national comprehensive health care reform, would have had minimal impact on specialized residential care for people with dementia. However, during the late 1990s, with the federal government shifting its focus to debt reduction and responding to pressures brought by the aging of the population, there will likely be significant changes in health care delivery and in the financing of public sector programs, including Medicare and Medicaid. These changes, in turn, portend major changes in special care programs.

The fate of Medicare will have little impact on dementia care, because Medicare primarily pays for acute care and rehabilitation. In fact, Medicaid and Supplemental Security Income are more directly tied to programs that support residents with dementia; changes in these payment systems could have a great impact on the care of these individuals.

Equally influential in this area will be the impact of market forces on special care programs. Part of the debate on health care reform in the early 1990s focused on the predictability of the health care budget through capitation. As a result of market forces rather than government initiative, managed care has taken over an ever-greater segment of the health care delivery system. Managed care and capitated programs under Medicare risk contracts have purposely left out long-term care coverage for older people. However, as these programs expand and have greater responsibility for the total care of older adults, including people with Alzheimer's disease, there will be changes in these programs to cover the care of people with dementia. Although they do not provide dementia-specific care, On-Lok and the PACE replications already offer evidence that merging funding streams can effectively lead to comprehensive coverage of the complete range of services required by older people with chronic illness.

Market forces will continue to play a key role in the development and evolution of special care programs, first in terms of controlling cost, and second, and most important, in terms of improving quality of care. Service providers who are and will be constantly looking for the best way to deliver care at the lowest cost will be pressured to maintain and expand market share as a strategy of competition. At the same time families will have increased expectations as to the type and level of care their family members receive. Thus, as consumers become more sophisticated, segments of the health care delivery system will become more sophisticated, leading to more options in special care programs. For example, in the mid-1990s the insurance industry improved the coverage offered under long-term care insurance plans, introducing products that covered multiple contingencies related to caring for people with Alzheimer's disease, including home care and skilled care. Low-cost options with minimal services are also likely to become more common in the marketplace, and these options may not best serve the needs of people with Alzheimer's disease.

Regardless of the efforts made by individual providers in the public and private sectors, a fundamental change has been occurring in the structure of long-term care: the increase in care management and the coordination of chronic care. What started as a mechanism to control costs will continue to evolve as a means of improving quality of care, including moving toward the development of a seamless continuum that serves people at all stages of Alzheimer's disease and other chronic impairments. This will be particularly efficacious for people with dementia, who move through the course of the disease at different rates, often presenting different symptoms. Just as the acute care system will continue to go through significant changes in order to provide alternative levels of care to best meet the needs of people with acute care needs, special care programs in residential settings will not be a monolithic service system. Starting with home- and community-based care, moving to multiple levels of residential services, and ultimately moving to late-stage care, delivery of services will be driven by outcomes. In addition, as clinical protocols and practice guidelines are implemented on a wider basis, the types of residents with dementia and their individual needs within special care programs will continue to evolve.

Another external influence on innovation and experimentation in the United States will be models of dementia care from other countries. The number of programs has grown significantly in the United States, and residential programs in Scandinavia, Western Europe, and the Pacific Rim have also expanded rapidly, often developing under regulatory and fiscal systems that differ from systems used in the United States. Many of the unique components and/or philosophies of these programs are gradually being introduced in the United States. As more information is disseminated regarding the effectiveness of these various programs, it is likely that innovation will come from outside as much as from within the United States.

The research community as well will continue to have an influence on the direction and development of special care programs. Primarily through federal research initiatives and grants, but also through philanthrophic and private efforts, researchers and clinicians are continuously experimenting with clinical strategies and modifications in service delivery interventions to identify the most effective programs to meet the needs of people with dementia. An increasing number of researchers are analyzing dementia-specific interventions and therapies (e.g., bathing, activities), changes in the physical environment (e.g., lighting), improvements in staff development (e.g., training protocols and methodologies), and program costs and financing. Combined with larger studies of changes in long-term service delivery and with studies specifically focusing on resident outcomes, researchers will increasingly look at the impact of changes in the health care system on special care programs. As Kane and others in the field have indicated, these initiatives are likely to lead to significant changes in types of special care programs and in the characteristics of residents in these settings, possibly leading to multiple levels of care based on the specific need for oversight of behavioral management and medical conditions of residents (Kane, 1994).

THE FUTURE

Dementia care is, and is destined to remain, a major consumer of health care resources for older people, at least until research identifies a cure or an intervention that can alter the process. Special care programs will hold a prominent position within the spectrum of services that will be necessary to care for the increasing number of people with dementia. Special care programs have emerged as the most sophisticated response to Alzheimer's disease. Whole fields of specialization have developed in architecture, interior design, nursing, and activities/recreation. Given the likelihood that dementia will be the preeminent health program of older people in the coming decades, special care programs can be expected to continue to grow.

The fact that research has failed to show dramatic differences between outcomes of specialized and integrated care settings has not slowed the expansion of special care programs. Other forces, such as finances, marketing, fashion, anecdotes, and testimonials, have had a far greater impact than research has on the direction of special care programs, which is often the case in the delivery of health services.

Because the forces that will shape the future of health care are shifting, the authors can only speculate on the future of special care programs. The following paragraphs comprise our best guesses on the changes that will occur from 1996 to 2016 (also see Table 12.3).

Table 12.3. Likely future changes in special care programs

Extension of specialization to all levels of care
Home care
Adult day services
Residential care/assisted living
Nursing facility home care
Hospice care
Greater emphasis on treatment and therapy
In physical design
In medical care (e.g., initiation and monitoring of medication)
Integration into managed care systems
More specific and less flexible regulation
In diagnosis and treatment of dementia
In design and function of special care programs
Special reimbursement for specialized care

Specialization will extend to all levels of care. Residential care (including assisted living), the most rapidly growing sector of specialized dementia care, will become a major provider of early- and mid-stage dementia care. Home health care agencies will develop specialized services for caregivers of people with dementia, and specialists in dementia will be on staff in all but the smallest of home health care agencies.

The emphasis on medical treatment and on alteration in functional outcomes will be greater. The majority of special care programs are largely custodial, and the majority of activities are social rather than therapeutic. As more medications become available, special care programs will need to be oriented more toward initiating, modifying, and monitoring medical treatment regimens. Concomitantly, more rigid protocols will exist for admission to special care programs (e.g., more accurate tests for Alzheimer's disease will be available). Functional outcomes will be monitored more closely, and, as a result, staff activities will be directed more toward treatments that make a difference functionally, such as prompted voiding and mobility programs.

Environmental design will focus more on treatment and less on marketing. The emphasis will be on products that promote safety, physical function, behavioral management, and orientation. These will include "smart" rooms, which automatically adjust lighting and alert staff when a resident with dementia gets up at night; soft, easy-to-clean, and odor-free floor surfaces; and better-designed appliances, such as chairs and bathtubs. Social trends toward a more humanistic environment will continue to have an effect on the design of special care programs, with more private rooms and with access to the outdoors and to aesthetic surroundings being encouraged to the extent that budgets allow.

Special care programs will be incorporated into integrated health care systems. Most health care for older people will likely be delivered within managed care systems. Special care programs for people with dementia will have a place within these systems to the extent that they provide more efficient and effective care. As is true of other areas of managed care, residents are likely to be moved more readily from one setting to another (i.e., in and out of specialized settings, depending on their needs at the time). Aging in place, which is common in many programs, will occur only in rural facilities or in facilities for poor people, unless it is clearly shown to cost less.

Regulation will increase with a resulting diminution in the diversity of settings and programs. Over time, a consensus will emerge as to when, how, and to whom specialized services should be delivered. This consensus will result in increased regulation and standardization. The source of these regulations will not always be the federal or state governments; managed care organizations will increasingly set their own internal standards. As a result, all facets of specialized care—the environment, staffing, nutritional programs, medical assessment/treatment, nursing care, and activities—are likely to be increasingly standardized. The result will be an overall increase in quality but a decrease in innovation.

Specialized units will be increasingly homogeneous. Long-term care will be increasingly owned and operated by large businesses and subject to standardization and regulation. Small and/or freestanding facilities, which have often been the greatest innovators and which have tended to do the best at containing costs, will be increasingly squeezed out. "McDonaldization" will occur in adult day services and residential care, as has already occurred in the nursing facility industry. Within this context, special care programs will look more and more alike.

Ethical dilemmas will remain a feature of dementia care, and special care programs will become increasingly versed in addressing them. Ethical quandaries will always be present in the care of people with terminal, progressive diseases, such as Alzheimer's disease. Technology merely reframes the questions; the issues are as old as human society. Thus, the future of dementia care will include the need to address issues of treatment goals and intensity. The staffs of special care programs will become increasingly expert at addressing these issues. In addition, managed care organizations and other third-party payers will increasingly dictate which treatments can be provided to whom.

Special reimbursement for special care programs will occur in some areas. The nursing facility industry has been singularly unsuccessful in convincing third-party payers that special care programs should have special reimbursement status. Private consumers have, however, been generally willing to pay extra for specialized care. Given the trend to restrict health care expenditures, it is likely that only certain specialized services will be approved for special reimbursement. For example, certain dementia-specific home health services are likely to be reimbursed, and if certain programs (e.g., mobility enhancement) can be shown to result in positive outcomes, special reimbursement is likely to be approved.

OUTCOME

Clearly the expansion of special care programs is inevitable, and their future will be influenced by multiple internal and external forces. As health care systems increasingly move to provide coverage for a full continuum of care in capitated environments, there will be increasing pressures to control costs while improving management of the care of people with dementia. Even greater interest in improving special care will come from the demand on the part of consumers to increase quality and improve the effectiveness of care. Underlying these pressures will be the limitations set by available public and private financing and our knowledge of best practices in Alzheimer's disease care. Although the knowledge of how to best provide specialized dementia care should improve significantly, the resources needed to offer this care are likely to be harder to come by as we move into the twenty-first century.

Still to come will be the influence of intangible changes in science and society. For example, along with the increasing success on the part of scientists who are trying to determine the genetic basis for Alzheimer's disease come complex ethical issues, such as how to deal with prospective identification of individuals who are predisposed to the disease and, thus, to using long-term care. The ethical quandary that these issues present to society inevitably leads to the question of how to best allocate improved special care programs in an era of shrinking resources.

Finally, while service providers and policy makers struggle to deal with the identification of best practices of residential care, the needs of individuals and families will constantly expand. It is these expanding consumer needs that will clearly set the tone and, ultimately, the level of responsiveness of the service provider community. As the course of special care programs changes they will need to be responsive to the needs of families and residents.

REFERENCES

Chandler, J.D., & Chandler, J.E. (1988). The prevalence of neuropsychiatric disorders in a nursing home population. *Journal of Geriatric Psychiatric Neurology, 1*, 71–76.

Coons, D. (1987). *Designing a residential care unit for persons with dementia*. Washington, DC: U.S. Office of Technology Assessment.

Evans, D. (1990). Estimated prevalence of Alzheimer's disease in the United States. *Milbank Quarterly, 68*, 267–289.

Kane, R. (1994). Harbingers of the future? Seeking the "special" in the dementia special care unit. *Alzheimer Disease & Associated Disorders, 8*(Suppl. 1), 425–428.

Kemper, P., & Murtaugh, C.M. (1991). Lifetime use of nursing home care. *New England Journal of Medicine, 324*(9), 595

Lair, T.J., & Lefkowitz, D.C. (1990). Mental health and functional status of residents of nursing and personal care homes. In *National Medical Expenditure Survey Research Findings* (DHHS Publication No. [PHS] 90-3470). Rockville, MD: Agency for Health Care Policy and Research, Public Health Service.

Maslow, K. (1994). Current knowledge about special care units: Findings of a study by the U.S. Office of Technology Assessment. *Alzheimer Disease & Associated Disorders, 8*(Suppl. 1), 14–40.

Office of Technology Assessment. (1987). *Losing a million minds: Confronting the tragedy of Alzheimer's disease and other dementias* (OTA-BA 323). Washington, DC: U.S. Government Printing Office.

Ory, M.G. (1994). Dementia special care: The development of a national research initiative. *Alzheimer's Disease & Associated Disorders, 8*(Suppl. 1), 389–394.

Rovner, B.W., German, P.S., Broadhead, J., Morris, R.K., Brant, L.J., Blaustein, J., & Folstein, M.F. (1990). The prevalence and management of dementia and other psychiatric disorders in nursing homes. *International Psychogeriatrics, 2*, 13–24.

Rovner, B.W., Kalfonek, S., & Filipp, L. (1986). Prevalence of mental illness in a community nursing home. *American Journal of Psychiatry, 143*, 1446–1449.

U.S. Department of Health and Human Services. (1991). *Mental illness in nursing homes: United States, 1985* (DHHS Publication No. [PHS] 91-1766). Rockville, MD: Author.

Volicer, L., Collard, A., Hurley, A., Bishop, C., Kern, D., & Karon, S. (1994). Impact of special care unit for patients with advanced Alzheimer's disease on patients' discomfort and costs. *Journal of the American Geriatrics Society, 42,* 597–603.

Supplemental Reading and Resources

Alzheimer's Disease Education and Referral Center (ADEAR). Information about Alzheimer's disease, diagnosis, treatment, and research.
ADEAR Center
Post Office Box 8250
Silver Spring, Maryland 20907-8250
Phone 800-438-4380
Fax 301-495-3334

Anderson, K.H., Hobson, A., Steiner, P., & Rodel, B. (1992). Patients with dementia: Involving families to maximize nursing care. *Journal of Gerontological Nursing, 12*(7), 19–24.

Beitler, D.G. (1993). Looking at special care units from a consumer's perspective. *Long-Term Care Quality Letter, 5*(20), 6–7.

Buckwalter, K.C., & Hall, G.R. (1987). Families of the institutionalized older adult: A neglected resource. In T.H. Brubaker (Ed.), *Aging, health, and family: Long term care* (pp. 176–196). Beverly Hills, CA: Sage Publications.

Cervantes, E., Heid-Grubman, J., & Schuerman, C.K. (1995). *The paraprofessional in home health and long-term care: Training modules for working with older adults.* Baltimore: Health Professions Press.

Cohen, D. (1994). Dementia, depression, and nutritional status. *Primary Care, 21*(1), 107–119.

Guidelines for dignity: Goals of specialized Alzheimer/dementia care in residential settings. (1992). Provides a framework for specialized care for people with dementia.
Alzheimer's Association
919 North Michigan Avenue, Suite 1000
Chicago, Illinois 60611-1676
800-272-3900

Gwyther, L.P. (1985). *Care of Alzheimer's patients: A manual for nursing home staff.* Chicago: Alzheimer's Disease and Related Disorders Association, Inc., and American Health Care Association.

Hall, G.R., & Buckwalter, K.C. (1987). Progressively lowered stress threshold: A conceptual model for care of adults with Alzheimer's disease. *Archives of Psychiatric Nursing, 1*(6), 306–309.

Hoffman, S.B., & Platt, C.A. (1991). *Comforting the confused: Strategies for managing dementia.* New York: Springer Publishing.

Linsk, N.L., Miller, B., Pflaum, R., & Ortigara-Vicik, A. (1988). Families, Alzheimer's disease, and nursing homes. *Journal of Applied Gerontology, 7,* 331–349.

Maas, M. (1988). The management of Alzheimer's disease patients in long term care facilities. *Nursing Clinics of North America, 23*(1), 57–68.

Maas, M., Buckwalter, K., Kelley, L., & Stolley, J. (1991). Family members' perceptions: How they view care of Alzheimer's patients in a nursing home. *Journal of Long-Term Care Administration, 19*(1), 21–25.

Mace, N. (1991). Dementia care units in nursing homes. In D.H. Coons (Ed.), *Specialized dementia care units* (pp. 55–82). Baltimore: The Johns Hopkins University Press.

McCracken, A. (1994). Special care units: Meeting the needs of cognitively impaired persons. *Journal of Gerontological Nursing, 20*(4), 41–46.

Mobily, P.R., Maas, M.L., Buckwalter, K.C., & Kelley, L.S. (1992). Staff stress on an Alzheimer's unit. *Journal of Psychosocial Nursing, 30*(9), 25–31.

Musson, N.D., Kincaid, J., Ryan, P., Glussman, B., Varone, L., Gammara, N., Wilson, R., Reese, W., & Silverman, M. (1990). Nature, nurture, nutrition: Interdisciplinary programs to address the prevention of malnutrition and dehydration. *Dysphagia, 5,* 96–101.

Residential settings: An examination of Alzheimer issues. (1994). Explores the current and future housing options for persons with dementia.
Alzheimer's Association
Patient and Family Services
919 North Michigan Avenue, Suite 1000
Chicago, Illinois 60611-1676
800-272-3900

Sloane, P.D., Lindeman, D.A., Phillips, C., Moritz, D.J., & Koch, G. (1995). Evaluating Alzheimer's special care units: Reviewing the evidence and identifying potential sources of bias. *Gerontologist, 35*(1), 103–111.

Springer, D., & Burbaker, T. (1984). *Family caregivers and dependent elderly.* Beverly Hills, CA: Sage Publications.

Standards and survey protocol for dementia special care units. (1994). Joint Commission on Accreditation of Healthcare Organizations standards, scoring guidelines, and explanations of their survey process to assess quality on dementia special care units.
Joint Commission on Accreditation of Healthcare Organizations
One Renaissance Boulevard
Oakbrook Terrace, Illinois 60181
708-916-5800

Volicer, L., Collard, A., Hurley, A., Bishop, C., & Karon, S. (1994). Impact of special care unit for patients with advanced Alzheimer's disease on patients' discomfort and costs. *Journal of the American Geriatrics Society, 42*, 597–603.

Walker, M.K., & Wekstein, D. (1990). *Nursing management of acutely ill elders with Alzheimer's disease.* Lexington: University of Kentucky.

Wilson, H.S. (1989). Family caregiving for a relative with Alzheimer's dementia: Coping with negative choices. *Nursing Research, 38*, 94–98.

Zinn, J.S., & Mor, V. (1994). Nursing home special care units: Distribution by type, state, and facility characteristics. *Gerontologist, 34*(3), 371–376.

Index

Page numbers followed by "f" indicate figures; page numbers followed by "t" indicate tables.

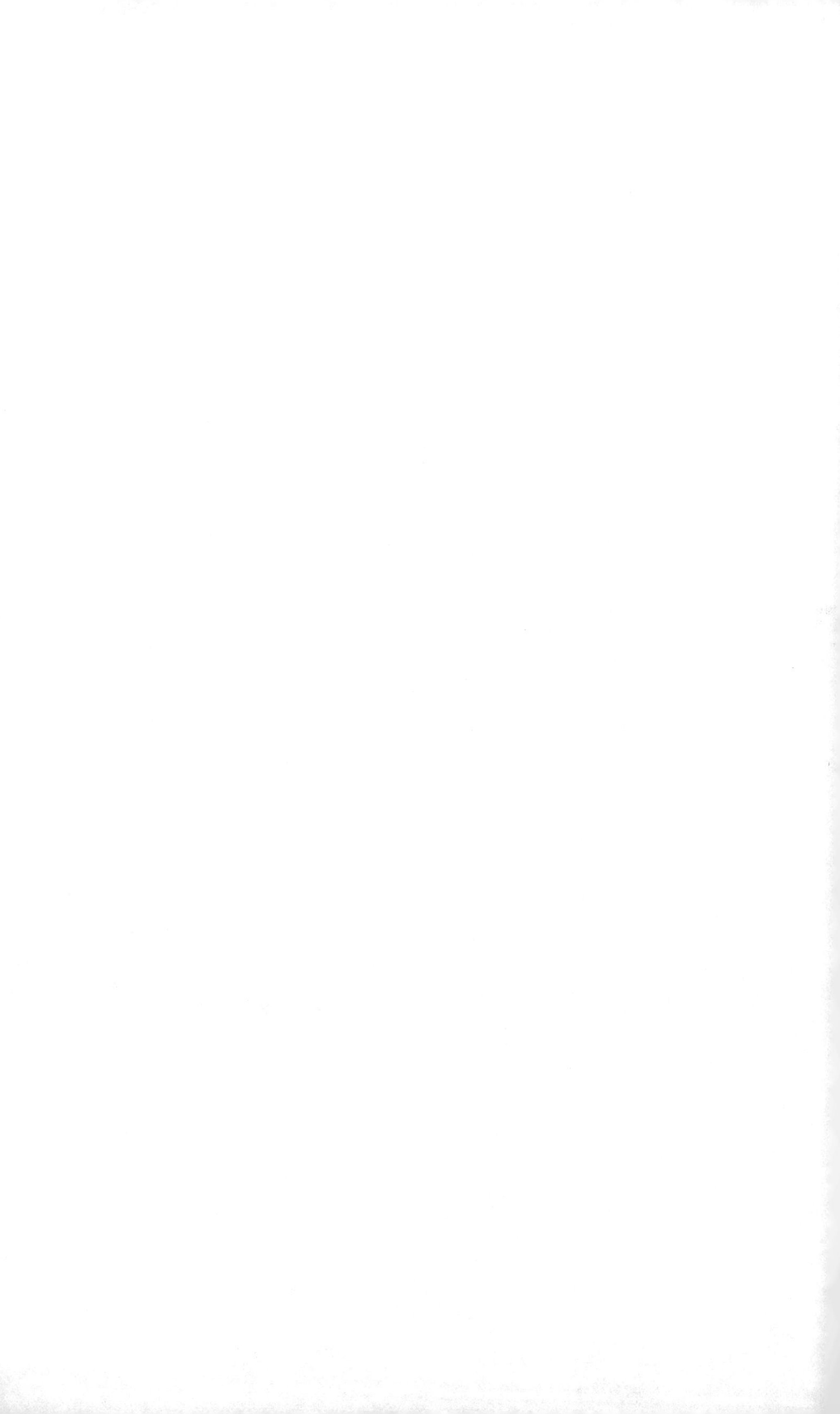